Official Journal of the International Pharmaco-EEG Society (IPEG)

Neuropsychobiology

International Journal of Experimental and Clinical Research in Biological Psychiatry, Pharmacopsychiatry, Biological Psychology/Pharmacopsychology and Pharmacoelectroencephalography

Founded 1975 by J. Mendlewicz (Brussels).
Since 1983 integrating 'International Pharmacopsychiatry',
founded 1968 by F.A. Freyhan (New York), N. Petrilowitsch (Mainz), P. Pichot (Paris)

KARGER

Printed in Switzerland on acid-free paper by Reinhardt Druck, Basel

Appears 6-weekly: 2 volumes per year (8 issues)

Guidelines for Authors

Neuropsychobiology

Submission

Only original papers written in English are considered and should be sent to the Editor of the corresponding section:

Biological Psychiatry

J. Mendlewicz
Université Libre de Bruxelles
Hôpital Erasme
Route de Lennik 808
B–1070 Bruxelles (Belgique)

Pharmacopsychiatry

B. Saletu
Allgemeines Krankenhaus
Universitätsklinik für Psychiatrie
Währinger Gürtel 18–20
A–1090 Wien (Österreich)

Biological Psychology/Pharmacopsychology

P. Netter
Justus-Liebig-Universität
Fachbereich 06, Psychologie
Otto-Behaghel-Strasse 10
D–35394 Giessen (Deutschland)

Pharmacoelectroencephalography

W.M. Herrmann
Freie Universität Berlin
Universitätsklinikum Benjamin Franklin
Psychiatrische Klinik und Poliklinik
Labor für Klinische Psychophysiologie
Eschenallee 3
D–14050 Berlin (Deutschland)

Manuscripts should be submitted in triplicate (with three sets of illustrations of which one is an original), typewritten double-spaced on one side of the paper, with a wide margin.

Conditions

All manuscripts are subject to editorial review. Manuscripts are received with the explicit understanding that they are not under simultaneous consideration by any other publication. Submission of an article for publication implies the transfer of the copyright from the author to the publisher upon acceptance. Accepted papers become the permanent property of 'Neuropsychobiology' and may not be reproduced by any means, in whole or in part, without the written consent of both the author and the publisher. It is the author's responsibility to obtain permission to reproduce illustrations, tables, etc. from other publications.

Arrangement

Title page: The first page of each paper should indicate the title, the authors' names, and the institute where the work was conducted. A short title for use as running head as well as the full address of the author to whom correspondence should be sent are also required.

Full address: The exact postal address complete with postal code must be given at the bottom of the title page. Please also supply phone and fax numbers, as well as your e-mail address.

Key words: For indexing purposes, a list of 3–10 key words in English is essential.

Abstract: Each paper needs an abstract of up to 10 lines.

Small type: Paragraphs which can or must be set in smaller type (case histories, test methods, etc.) should be indicated with a 'p' (petit) in the margin on the left-hand side.

Footnotes: Avoid footnotes. When essential, they are numbered consecutively and typed at the foot of the appropriate page.

Tables and illustrations: Tables and illustrations (both numbered in Arabic numerals) should be prepared on separate sheets. Tables require a heading and figures a legend, also prepared on a separate sheet. For the reproduction of illustrations, only good drawings and original photographs can be accepted; negatives or photocopies cannot be used. Due to technical reasons, figures with a screen background should not be submitted. When possible, group several illustrations on one block for reproduction (max. size 181 × 223 mm) or provide crop marks. On the back of each illustration, indicate its number, the author's name, and 'top' with a soft pencil.

Color illustrations: Up to 6 color illustrations per page can be integrated within the text at the reduced price of CHF 660.– / USD 545.00 per page. Color illustrations are reproduced at the author's expense.

References: In the text identify references by Arabic numerals [in square brackets]. Material submitted for publication but not yet accepted should be noted as 'unpublished data' and not be included in the reference list. The list of references should include only those publications which are cited in the text. Do not alphabetize; number references in the order in which they are first mentioned in the text. The surnames of the authors followed by initials should be given. There should be no punctuation other than a comma to separate the authors. Cite all authors, 'et al' is not sufficient. Abbreviate journal names according to the Index Medicus system. (Also see International Committee of Medical Journal Editors: Uniform requirements for manuscripts submitted to biomedical journals. N Engl J Med 1997;336:309–315.)

Examples
(a) Papers published in periodicals: Sun J, Koto H, Chung KF: Interaction of ozone and allergen challenges on bronchial responsiveness and inflammation in sensitised guinea pigs. Int Arch Allergy Immunol 1997;112:191–195.
(b) Monographs: Matthews DE, Farewell VT: Using and Understanding Medical Statistics, ed 3, revised. Basel, Karger, 1996.
(c) Edited books: Parren PWHI, Burton DR: Antibodies against HIV-1 from phage display libraries: Mapping of an immune response and progress towards antiviral immunotherapy; in Capra JD (ed): Antibody Engineering. Chem Immunol. Basel, Karger, 1997, vol 65, pp 18–56.

Page charges

There are no page charges for papers of 4 or fewer printed pages (including tables, illustrations and references). Each additional complete or partial page is charged to the author at CHF 275.– / USD 196.00. The allotted size of a paper is equal to approx. 12 manuscript pages (including tables, illustrations and references).

Galley proofs

Unless indicated otherwise, galley proofs are sent to the first-named author and should be returned with the least possible delay. Alterations made in galley proofs, other than the correction of printer's errors, are charged to the author. No page proofs are supplied.

Reprints

Order forms and a price list are sent with the galley proofs. Orders submitted after the issue is printed are subject to considerably higher prices.

Methodology

The methodology section may be set in small print.

Subjects: The total number of subjects (or animals) included in a study should be given.
The number of dropouts and the reason for dropping out should be indicated. In addition to a valid case analysis, an intent-to-treat analysis should usually be done. The criteria for selecting subjects should be given. The type of subjects, both volunteers and patients, should be described in detail; the therapeutic milieu should be mentioned.

KARGER

Fax +41 61 306 12 34
E-Mail karger@karger.ch
www.karger.com

The Guidelines for Authors are available at:
www.karger.com/journals/nps/nps_gl.htm

Methods: All methods and variables used in the trial should be described. If all the variables are not reported in the paper presented, this should be indicated. For each method and variable, either a detailed description including aspects of reliability and validity and/or an adequate reference should be given. If at all possible a placebo group should be included in trials.

EEG-Methods: If EEG or EP/ERP data are presented, the Guidelines for Experimental Designs, Data Acquisition and EEG-Mapping and/or currently issued guidelines of IPEG should be taken into account.

Data presentation: The data presentation should enable a reader to understand the results from the data to a maximum extent. If single values are not presented, means, standard deviations, type of statistics used (e.g. F, t, χ^2 and p values, two-tailed) should be given. For nominal or ordinal data, frequency tables are applicable (absolute values, percentages).

Biometrics and statistics: In the case of drug studies, the type of study (e.g. phase I, early or late phase II, phase III or IV) and the aim should be clearly defined. It is of relevance whether a study is performed to end up with a hypothesis or if it is performed to test existing hypotheses. The statistical procedure, including the statistical model and the underlying assumptions should be presented. If more than one statistical method is used for primary outcome variables, the reasons should be indicated.
It should be stated clearly whether exploratory descriptive or confirmatory data analyses are done. If more than one outcome variable is used, the study protocol should clearly discriminate between primary target variables and secondary (descriptive) variables.
If confirmatory statistics are done (e.g. in a phase III drug trial to prove efficacy), then the test strategy to avoid an inflation of the type I error (α) has to be clearly indicated. If a comparison to a standard drug is done, the type II error (β) in relation to the differences has to be taken into consideration.

Clinical relevance: The study planning, including the biometrical planning, should be done in a way that any clinically relevant differences can be detected by the study. The statistical methods should be described.

Rater and interrater training: The type, qualification and experience of the rater should be indicated. If more than one rater was involved in one rating, it has to be indicated how interrater reliability was ensured. This is of special importance if studies are done in more than one ward of a hospital or center or as multicenter trials.

GLP or GCP: It has to be indicated whether the animal trial has been done in accordance with good laboratory practice and in case of a clinical trial whether the rules of good clinical practice were respected. The type of monitoring, auditing and source data verification should be indicated.

Ethics: Ethical considerations, benefits and risks of a trial must be mentioned: in addition, it has to be indicated how informed consent was obtained.

General Information

Neuropsychobiology

Publication data: 'Neuropsychobiology' is published 8 times a year. Volumes 41–42, each with 4 issues, appear in 2000.

Subscription rates: Subscriptions run for a full calendar year. Prices are given per volume.
Personal subscription:
Subscription + postage and handling
CHF 276.– + CHF 17.30 Europe
CHF 276.– + CHF 26.10 Overseas
USD 211.00 + USD 17.30
(Must be in the name of, billed to, and paid by an individual. Order must be marked 'personal subscription'.)
Institutional subscription:
Subscription + postage and handling
CHF 552.– + CHF 21.60 Europe
CHF 552.– + CHF 32.60 Overseas
USD 422.00 + USD 21.60
Airmail postage: CHF 24.–, USD 20.00.
(Extra per volume.)
Discount subscription prices:
Ass. Eur. Psych.; Int. Pharmaco-EEG Society (IPEG); APA; Interdisc. Soc. Biol. Psych.

Advertising: Correspondence and rate requests should be addressed to the Publisher.

Microforms: Please direct all enquiries and orders to: University Microfilms Inc.
300 North Zeeb Road, P.O. Box 1346
Ann Arbor, MI 48106-1346 (USA)

Subscription orders: Orders can be placed at agencies, bookstores, directly with the Publisher
S. Karger AG, P.O. Box,
CH–4009 Basel (Switzerland)
or with any of the following distributors:
Deutschland: S. Karger GmbH, Postfach
D–79095 Freiburg
France: Librairie Luginbühl
36, bd de Latour-Maubourg, F–75007 Paris
Great Britain, Ireland: S. Karger Publishers
58 Grove Hill Road
Tunbridge Wells, Kent TN1 1SP
USA: S. Karger Publishers, Inc.
26 West Avon Road, P.O. Box 529
Farmington, CT 06085
India, Bangladesh, Sri Lanka:
S. Karger India Subscription Agency
B–5/132 Safdarjung Enclave
New Delhi-110029
Japan: Katakura Libri, Inc.
2F, Marushima Bldg, 4-6-17, Yushima,
Bunkyo-ku, Tokyo 113-0034

Change of address: Both old and new address should be sent to the subscription source.

Single issues and back volumes: Information can be obtained through the Publisher.

Bibliographic indices: This journal is regularly listed in bibliographic services, including Current Contents®.

Book Reviews: Books are accepted for review by special agreement.

Fax+ 41 61 306 12 34
E-Mail karger@karger.ch
www.karger.com

The Journal Home Page is available at:
www.karger.com/journals/nps

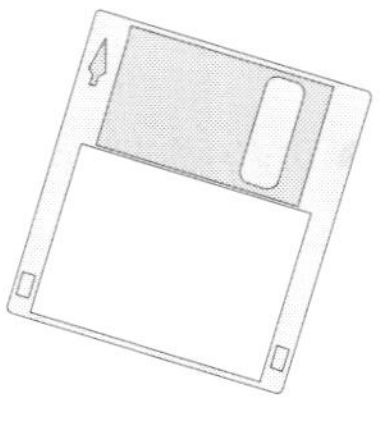

Disk Submission

A **comprehensive version** of these guidelines for the **submission of manuscripts and illustrations on disk** can be accessed online under **www.karger.com/journals/disksub.htm** or requested as a leaflet from the editorial department.

Please follow the general rules on style and arrangement in the **"Guidelines for Authors"** of the journal. Submit a **double-spaced printout** of your manuscript matching the file on disk exactly.

Technical Information
Store only data pertinent to this manuscript. Include your fonts (screen and printer fonts for Macintosh).
For a **text only** manuscript, use a 3.5 inch disk.
For **text and illustrations,** use 3.5 or 5.25 Magneto Optical Disc; CD-ROM (DOS or hybrid); iomage Zip/DOS (100 MB), or 44 MB, 88 MB or 200 MB SyQuest. Compress extensive data using ZIP format.

Data Description
Label your disk with the **title of the journal or book** for which it is submitted; a **short version** of the paper's title; your **name,** postal and e-mail address, fax and phone number; **hard and software** used, including the version; and the **complete list of the file names.** File names consist of eight characters before the dot identifying the file and three characters after the dot identifying the application.

Text and Format
The **preferred word-processing package is MS-Word.** Other commonly used PC text programs and ASCII formats are accepted.
Update your data when you revise subsequent to the reviewer's or editor's decision and mark revisions clearly. Manuscripts accepted for publication are subject to **copy editing:** changes and/or questions will be marked in the manuscript, which will be returned to you with your disk and the galley proofs for checking.
Enter your text continuously flush left. Do not use any layout functions. Do not split words at the end of a line. **Do not use indentations.** Use a blank line before and a hard return at the end of paragraphs.
Arrange headings flush left. Insert only **one space after punctuation marks.** Insert Greek letters, mathematical symbols etc. with your word-processing program. Use **boldface and italics** as well as sub- and superscript where appropriate.
Tables are part of the text and should be placed at the end of the text file. Separate the individual parts of a table by lines. Use the tabulator instead of spaces. Format operation data on one line in the same column. **Legends to illustrations are part of the text** and should also be listed at the end of the text file.

Illustrations
Store illustrations as separate files: do not embed them in your text. Export **line drawings/vector graphics** as TIF, EPS or WMF format. Use Photoshop for processing and retouching **scanned halftone images.** Save the original scan and the processed version. Export **black and white or color images** as TIF or EPS format in their anticipated size in print. **For detailed information** on how to submit illustration data on disk please consult the leaflet or **www.karger.com/journals/disksub.htm.**

KI 98 DISK

KARGER

Fax + 41 61 306 12 34
E-Mail karger@karger.ch
www.karger.com

The Guidelines for Authors are available at:
www.karger.com/journals/nps

Neuropsychobiology

Traits as Dispositions for Psychopathology

Symposium 'Traits as Dispositions for Psychopathology'
September 27–October 1, 1998, Dresden, Germany

Editors
Petra Netter, Giessen
Burkhard Brocke, Dresden

10 figures and 6 tables, 2000

All papers have undergone the Journal's usual peer review

KARGER
Basel · Freiburg · Paris · London · New York ·
New Delhi · Bangkok · Singapore · Tokyo · Sydney

S. Karger
Medical and Scientific Publishers
Basel · Freiburg · Paris · London
New York · New Delhi · Bangkok
Singapore · Tokyo · Sydney

Drug Dosage
The authors and the publisher have exerted every effort to ensure that drug selection and dosage set forth in this text are in accord with current recommendations and practice at the time of publication. However, in view of ongoing research, changes in government regulations, and the constant flow of information relating to drug therapy and drug reactions, the reader is urged to check the package insert for each drug for any change in indications and dosage and for added warnings and precautions. This is particularly important when the recommended agent is a new and/or infrequently employed drug.

Printed in Switzerland on acid-free paper by
Reinhardt Druck, Basel
ISBN 3–8055–6911–4

KARGER

Fax+ 41 61 306 12 34
E-Mail karger@karger.ch
www.karger.com

Vol. 41, No 1, 2000

Neuropsychobiology

Contents

KARGER

Fax+41 61 306 12 34
E-Mail karger@karger.ch
www.karger.com

Access to full text and tables of contents, including tentative ones for forthcoming issues: www.karger.com/journals/nps/nps_bk.htm

Neuropsychobiology

Neuropsychobiology 2000;41:5–23

Six Basic Dimensions of Personality and a Seventh Factor of Generalized Dysfunctional Personality: A Diathesis System Covering all Personality Disorders

Burghard Andresen

Psychiatric Clinic, University Hospital Hamburg-Eppendorf, Hamburg, Germany

Key Words

Personality disorder · Five-factor model · Cognitive aberration · Factor analysis · Diathesis model

Abstract

The five-factor model (FFM) of personality has recently been claimed to be comprehensive for all dimensionally conceived personality disorders (PDs). This assumption is refuted on the grounds of a principal component analysis conducted for three basic factor inventories (FFPI, NEO-FFI, Hamburg Personality Inventory), 22 explorative facet scales for normal personality and a questionnaire inventory (Inventory of Clinical Personality Accentuations) of 24 PD scales. Seven substantial orthogonal Varimax factors were found explaining 73% of the total variance. The five factors of the FFM were replicated. In addition, a new basic factor 'risk and competition seeking' (basic dimension 'risk', BD-R) emerged replicating findings of Andresen. The massive seventh factor was substantially loaded by all 24 PD scales and interpreted as 'general dysfunctional personality' (GDP). Most of the highly loaded scales describe varying forms of cognitive aberration. Together with GDP, the six-factor model now explains about 73% of all PD scales, thus, a virtually comprehensive descriptive diathesis system is achieved. Without GDP and BD-R, only 25% can be accounted for by the FFM. Five of the six normal dimensions will be loaded with positive and negative signs by some PDs. Neuroticism (BD-N) is still unique regarding its positive substantial correlations with almost all PD scales. BD-N is also the only normal factor which is correlated with GDP at about 0.50. A geometric model for the relationships between basic and clinical factors is presented.

Introduction

Recent research on structural relations between personality disorders (PDs) and normal basic dimensions of personality [1] was mainly guided by the 'five-factor model' (FFM), a concept of five comprehensive, orthogonal and culturally invariant second-order dimensions of all central personality descriptors [2, 3]. Several advocates of this model – which still remains hypothetical and controversially discussed in all its claims and promises [4–10] – hypothesized that the 'big five' may sufficiently explain all personality disturbances on the dimensional level [1, 11–13]. This conviction stems from some earlier empirical studies in this field [14–19].

KARGER

Fax + 41 61 306 12 34
E-Mail karger@karger.ch
www.karger.com

0302–282X/00/0411–0005$17.50/0

Accessible online at:
www.karger.com/journals/nps

PD Dr. Burghard Andresen, PhD
University Clinic Hamburg-Eppendorf
Clinic for Psychiatry and Psychotherapy
Martinistrasse 52, D–20246 Hamburg (Germany)
Tel. +49 40 42803 4214, Fax +49 4539 891416

This hypothesis – see also the representative handbook by Costa and Widiger [20] – led to the proposal that the FFM and its prominent diagnostic instruments could replace the psychiatric categorial DSM PD system or be a superior dimensional alternative [21]. In rather sharp contrast to this forceful approach, the latest revision of the DSM-IV [22] put a preliminary end to this 'replacement discussion'. It is important to underline that no definite dimensional research criteria, not even in the DSM-IV addendum, were established, although even for the most prominent psychiatric disease – schizophrenia – a three-dimensional diagnostic approach [23] has already been introduced as a reasonable conceptual alternative to the well-established typological subdivision of this disorder.

Correlational Evidence of Relations between FFM and PD Scales

Actually, the rather bold idea about the axis II comprehensiveness of the big five presented in the late eighties and early nineties was never convincingly demonstrated on empirical grounds. Methodologically advanced studies which separated normal and clinical dimensions in terms of regression approaches [18, 24–28] showed that the correlational predictive power of the FFM dimensions was much too low to favor the early claims. Mean R^2 values are presented in a range of 0.15–0.45 if questionnaire-questionnaire comparisons are made. If clinical PD syndromes are assessed by interview, the typical R^2 levels are much lower (0.15–0.25). With due caution and applying approximate corrections for inconsistency of scales it can be said that about 50% of reliable PD scale variance is not explained by the FFM in the typical study of this kind, where questionnaires with questionnaire subscales are correlated on both sides without method variance leading to attenuation effects.

Most explanatory power is given for the dimensions of neuroticism (basic dimension 'neuroticism', BD-N). BD-N is regularly correlated in the same positive direction with almost all PD scales. According to McCrae [11], high scores on BD-N will be present in practically all PDs, while combinations of traits on the other four dimensions should determine the type of PD.

Agreeableness (BD-A) is also quite strong regarding its rather uniform negative predictive quality for most PDs. Extraversion (BD-E) has been moderately predictive in some studies showing rather strong positive and negative correlations with different PD scales. Openness to experience (BD-O) has no strong correlations with any PD scale. Conscientiousness (BD-C) also is quite inefficient in predicting PDs.

Reviewing these empirical data, the statement of Davis and Millon [29] seems to be justified that there is only 'partial overlap between these two universes of discourse' and that for PDs there must be a distinctive contribution from dimensional concepts or other sources beyond the big five.

Some experts would argue that the clinical scales in these studies are of lower hierarchical position in the FFM and therefore only for this reason far below the optimum of prediction (mismatch of hierarchical levels), but the evidence in favor of this objection is very poor [14, 28, 30].

Thus, a conclusion from these studies would be that FFM instruments can replace neither specific clinical PD interviews nor PD questionnaires to operationalize PDs on the dimensional level. Thus, the DSM-IV task force was right to refute the proposal mentioned above. This of course does not mean that categorial systems are generally superior to dimensional ones [31], quite the reverse seems to be true. It just means that the normal FFM inventories cannot be a reasonable alternative to dimensional questionnaire PD description with direct criterion-based validity.

How to Optimize PD Prediction from a Basic Dimensional System

Searching for more powerful explanations of clinical PD scales based on a theoretically founded, invariant second-order structure of near orthogonal personality dimensions remains a prominent and valuable goal for many practical and theoretical reasons. How could such enhancements be achieved?

Other Systems of Normal Dimensions Might be More Efficient in PD Prediction

The available knowledge about this possibility [32–37] shall not be discussed in detail. There is no convincing evidence that changing the system of basic personality dimensions would result in more substantial prediction of PD scales, but empirical research on this question is too limited to definitely exclude this possibility.

Other and Extended Systems of PDs May Be Closer to the Normal Dimensions

A low statistical relationship between normal and clinical dimensions may also depend on unrepresentative sampling of PD concepts in the currently favored DSM system. Duijsens and Diekstra [27] did not find differences in big five predictability between ICD-10 and DSM-III-R PD scales. But the question goes far beyond this. Westen and Arkowitz-Westen [38] also presented evidence that even practitioners in the psychiatric field may favor quite different concepts compared to the established official diagnostic categories.

In this context, the question arises why the recently best replicated factorial structures of PDs are only three- or four-dimensional [37, 39–43] and do not show an approximate 1:1 correspondence with the FFM (not even on a low correlational level). And why should BD-O not come out with a sufficiently clear and substantial pattern of PD correlations? These mismatches may be interpreted as evidence for severe unrepresentative sampling of PD criteria and scales which has to be overcome. Widiger and Costa [1], for instance, mention 'alexithymia' as a potential PD with strong negative correlations to BD-O.

For these and several other reasons, future research should also explore quite different concepts of PDs not included in the DSM-IV and ICD-10.

More Basic Normal Factors Should Give Better Prediction

Of course, adding further orthogonal basic dimensions to the FFM, if they exist, could enhance the predictive power of normal personality dimensions towards PD scales. Several proposals and scales have been presented for normal dimensions beyond or in addition to the big five [6, 7, 10, 44–47]. A replicated incremental effect on PD scale prediction has until now only been demonstrated by Andresen [9, 48], who proposed a sixth basic factor of 'risk and competition seeking' (BD-R) with additional negative predictive relevance for all anxious-fearful PD scales and positive relevance for all antisocial, risking and behaviorally expansive aspects of PDs. Nevertheless, these incremental effects are only moderate in size.

Addition of a Cognitive Aberrant Personality Factor

Costa and McCrae [15, 49] discuss the existence of a sixth 'cognitive aberration' factor beyond the FFM which can explain a considerable proportion of PD scale variance. Wiggins and Pincus [14] indeed found a fifth factor of PDs with loadings of scales for schizotypal and paranoid PD besides a four-factor system resembling the empirical solutions mentioned above. This PD factor is – in contrast to the other four PD factors which show maximal correlations with FFM scales between 0.53 and 0.71 – not substantially correlated with the FFM factors. With $r = 0.27$ only BD-N shows some shared variance. BD-O surprisingly correlates with this psychosis proneness factor only by 0.12. In some respects such a dimension reminds us of the early conception of a basic 'psychoticism' factor proposed by Eysenck and Eysenck [50]. The revised version published much later [51], however, is too negatively correlated with the normal BD-C and BD-A factors of the FFM [52] to be accepted as a basic psychopathological PD dimension beyond the big five. Substantial correlations of the revised variant with schizotypy measures could not be found [53, 54]. However, the early psychoticism factor – more correlated with BD-N and therefore revised – was very 'psychosis prone' or 'psychotic like' and had the schizotypal and paranoid qualities of the fifth factor of Wiggins and Pincus [14]. In other reviews, Costa and McCrae [49] made a drawback from such assumptions regarding a sixth cognitive aberration factor which would give up the claim of FFM being comprehensive for all PDs.

Introducing a basic dimension of cognitive aberration is of course a qualitative step in model building. The core psychopathological features of some clearly dysfunctional PDs would be incorporated into the explanatory model, at least at the dimensional level. In adding this clinical dimension, the basic factor model for strictly normal traits is definitely violated. But it should be kept in mind that FFM advocates claim that their model is comprehensive for the total personality sphere including PDs [1], thus also implicitly giving up the dimensional distinction between normal and abnormal. The difference is therefore: assuming a central psychopathology factor in addition to a five or five + x set of normal dimensions leads to a dual system, where severe forms of disorder with dysfunctional and especially cognitive aberration contents are 'collected' by one factor, and the other factors, namely NR, are more or less 'cleaned' from these clinical aspects.

Furthermore, such a model, incorporating psychosis prone maladjustment of personality, is open to criticism regarding axis I spectrum disorders which according to some authors belong to the axis I psychiatric field and should per se not be integrated into the personality sphere. This also is the position of the International Classification of Disease, 10th revision (ICD-10) [55]. In the ICD-10, spectrum personality concepts appear in modified form under the respective sections of axis I disorders. Therefore the 'schizotypal syndrome' shows up in altered 'makeup' under F2 reserved for schizophrenic and delusional/paranoid disorders. Especially the schizotypal personality syndrome is up to now a construct 'between the two worlds', axis I and II [54]. On the other hand, schizotypal or paranoid PDs have been stable units of DSM-IV PD diagnosis for a long time, and therefore, the rigid argument against spectrum constructs because of overlapping relevance also for axis I attacks the well-established DSM categorization of PDs.

Table 1. Varimax loadings with variance fractionations for seven factors of an 8-FS derived from a PC factor analysis of 62 personality scales

Scale	GDP	NR	EX	OE	CO	AG	RC	MV stat.	EV GDP	EV SFM	EV 7 fac.	CA
ICP-G-STY schizotypal	*0.80*	0.15	0.03	0.13	−0.06	0.03	0.30	*3*	64.2	13.2	77.4	0.88
ICP-E-OTY obsessiotypal	*0.79*	0.23	−0.08	0.05	0.02	0.03	0.07	*3*	63.2	7.0	70.2	0.91
ICP-G-NEG negativistic	*0.76*	0.26	−0.18	−0.13	0.08	−0.11	0.24	*3*	58.5	19.9	78.4	0.89
ICP-E-ANX anxious	*0.73*	0.29	−0.16	−0.02	−0.14	0.05	−0.26	*2*	53.7	19.8	73.5	0.91
ICP-E-DIS dissociative	*0.73*	0.14	0.01	0.25	−0.26	0.03	0.22	*2*	53.4	19.9	73.3	0.90
ICP-E-AST asthenic	*0.68*	*0.40*	−0.06	0.07	0.01	0.04	−0.05	*1*	45.8	17.5	63.3	0.91
ICP-G-PAR paranoid	*0.68*	0.14	−0.09	−0.16	0.28	−0.13	*0.34*	*2*	45.7	26.7	72.4	0.89
ICP-G-DEP dependent	*0.66*	0.13	−0.04	−0.26	0.06	0.02	−0.05	*2*	44.1	9.3	53.4	0.89
ICP-G-BOR borderline	*0.66*	*0.42*	0.02	0.06	−0.28	−0.21	0.20	*1*	43.4	34.8	78.2	0.90
ICP-G-PHO phobic (phys.)	*0.65*	0.08	0.02	0.03	0.26	−0.09	*−0.50*	0	41.9	33.6	75.5	0.83
ICP-P-REG regressive	*0.63*	0.26	0.07	*0.45*	*−0.31*	0.06	0.21	0	39.2	41.9	81.1	0.85
ICP-P-HAV harm avoid.	*0.62*	0.13	−0.13	−0.09	0.26	0.20	*−0.36*	*1*	37.9	28.0	65.9	0.74
ICP-E-EXP explosive	*0.59*	*0.44*	0.19	−0.08	−0.13	−0.21	0.14	0	34.6	31.6	66.2	0.91
ICP-G-SCH schizoid	*0.56*	0.20	*−0.55*	−0.05	−0.02	−0.22	0.26	0	31.7	45.9	77.6	0.90
ICP-G-HIS histrionic	*0.56*	0.17	*0.52*	0.16	−0.08	−0.16	0.27	0	31.5	43.2	74.7	0.87
ICP-G-SAV soc. avoidant	*0.56*	0.19	*−0.60*	−0.06	0.02	−0.04	−0.10	0	31.4	41.9	73.3	0.91
ICP-P-STR stress prone	*0.54*	*0.67*	−0.05	0.16	−0.09	0.03	−0.21	0	28.8	53.6	82.4	0.90
ICP-P-FEA fearful-tender	*0.54*	0.19	0.10	0.11	0.19	0.06	*−0.64*	0	28.6	50.3	78.9	0.86
ICP-G-DPR depressive	*0.53*	*0.55*	*−0.38*	0.03	−0.11	−0.06	0.11	0	28.5	47.2	75.7	0.91
ICP-G-ANT antisocial	*0.53*	0.03	0.06	−0.09	−0.13	*−0.49*	*0.48*	0	27.8	50.5	78.3	0.88
ICP-G-COM compulsive	*0.53*	0.00	−0.22	−0.18	*0.58*	0.07	0.13	0	27.8	43.4	71.2	0.85
ICP-G-NAR narcissistic	*0.52*	−0.04	0.16	0.22	0.10	−0.30	*0.49*	0	27.5	42.1	69.6	0.90
ICP-P-ALE alexithymic	*0.44*	−0.02	−0.24	*−0.57*	0.24	*−0.32*	0.17	0	19.1	56.3	75.4	0.76
ICP-P-OPP oppositional	*0.39*	*0.35*	−0.13	−0.01	0.10	*−0.52*	*0.36*	0	15.6	54.7	80.3	0.87
HPI-D-N sensible	*0.52*	*0.73*	−0.05	0.11	0.01	−0.06	−0.02	0	27.6	54.7	82.3	0.92
FFPI-ES(-) emot. unstable	*0.46*	*0.64*	−0.16	0.04	−0.14	−0.04	−0.27	0	20.9	53.3	74.2	0.88
NEO-FFI-N neurotic	*0.51*	*0.65*	−0.15	0.08	−0.10	0.07	−0.23	0	26.2	51.4	77.6	0.86
HPI-F-STA stable	−0.27	*−0.77*	0.05	−0.04	0.18	0.11	0.27	*3*	7.0	71.7	78.7	0.84
HPI-F-CON contented	−0.24	*−0.78*	0.17	0.07	0.12	0.04	0.05	*3*	5.6	66.6	72.2	0.73
HPI-F-OPT optimistic	−0.09	*−0.63*	*0.52*	0.03	0.12	0.16	0.16	0	0.9	73.7	74.6	0.82
HPI-D-E extraverted	0.02	−0.05	*0.86*	0.04	−0.02	0.14	0.28	*3*	0.0	84.0	84.0	0.92
FFPI-E extraverted	−0.23	−0.18	*0.87*	−0.03	−0.06	0.08	0.04	*3*	5.2	79.4	84.6	0.89
NEO-FFI-E extraverted	−0.09	−0.21	*0.82*	0.04	−0.02	0.05	0.17	*3*	0.9	75.3	76.2	0.78
HPI-F-SOL solitary	0.20	0.02	*−0.81*	−0.03	0.12	−0.06	0.01	*3*	3.9	67.6	71.5	0.84
HPI-F-SUR surgent	0.06	−0.15	*0.75*	0.08	−0.06	−0.02	*0.44*	*1*	0.3	78.6	78.9	0.84
HPI-F-SES entertai. seek.	0.08	0.13	*0.43*	0.14	0.14	−0.05	*0.38*	0	0.7	38.1	38.8	0.68

Aims of the Study

This work is principally directed at all these questions and especially at the last one, but of course it cannot explore all ways and options empirically. As a result of literature studies and several own empirical works [7–9], the author tries to establish a new basic dimensional model of truly parsimonious and comprehensive personality description including all PD concepts.

These model-building aspects shall be exemplified by a large-scale dimensional analysis of 62 normal and clinical personality scales covering an extended range of traits and syndromes. This approach is descriptive, based solely on an explorative principal component analysis with subsequent Varimax rotation. Strong emphasis is laid on comprehensiveness and fractionation of explained variance. Consequences for neuropsychobiological and especially genetic personality research will be discussed.

Method

Subjects

Three hundred and ninety-five subjects participated in this study (210 were female, 185 male; mean age 33.6, SD 12.6). Educational status covered a wide range with a slight bias towards higher education. Exclusion criteria regarding psychiatric, psychosomatic or somatic disorders were not used, thus, diverse sources and different amounts of (psycho)pathology may have influenced the results to the degree that will be present in unselected normal populations.

Table 1 (continued)

Scale	GDP	NR	EX	OE	CO	AG	RC	MV stat.	EV GDP	EV SFM	EV 7 fac.	CA
HPI-D-O alternative or.	0.11	0.07	0.06	*0.83*	–0.18	0.20	0.21	*3*	1.2	80.7	81.9	0.89
FFPI-IA independent	*–0.36*	–0.18	*0.32*	0.23	0.10	–0.05	*0.37*	0	12.7	33.9	46.6	0.87
NEO-FFI-O open to exper.	–0.12	0.00	0.02	*0.77*	–0.21	0.11	0.14	*3*	1.3	67.7	69.0	0.74
HPI-F-REF reflective	0.22	0.01	0.10	*0.69*	–0.15	*0.38*	–0.02	*1*	4.7	66.4	71.1	0.85
HPI-F-VIS visionary	0.25	0.08	0.23	*0.48*	–0.13	–0.08	*0.54*	0	6.1	60.3	66.4	0.79
HPI-F-ERO ero. exp. seek.	0.14	0.04	*0.67*	*0.42*	–0.01	0.05	0.27	*1*	2.0	71.1	73.1	0.83
HPI-F-INT intelligent	–0.06	–0.03	0.21	*0.36*	*0.35*	–0.20	*0.48*	0	0.4	56.6	57.0	0.91
HPI-D-C normative or.	0.03	–0.12	–0.05	–0.18	*0.87*	0.14	0.17	*3*	0.1	85.3	85.4	0.90
FFPI-C conscientious	–0.25	–0.16	–0.12	–0.17	*0.76*	0.14	–0.22	*3*	6.5	73.0	79.5	0.87
NEO-FFI-C conscientious	–0.24	–0.22	0.03	–0.05	*0.79*	0.07	0.03	*3*	5.9	67.7	73.6	0.84
HPI-F-PER persistent	0.09	–0.10	0.16	–0.13	*0.64*	–0.03	*0.49*	0	0.8	70.9	71.7	0.75
HPI-F-CSV conservative	0.24	–0.04	–0.13	*–0.51*	*0.64*	–0.02	0.07	0	6.0	69.7	75.7	0.85
HPI-F-TRA traditional	0.08	0.00	0.02	–0.12	*0.50*	*0.54*	0.08	0	0.6	56.8	57.4	0.67
HPI-D-A altruistic	0.15	0.03	0.20	0.22	0.14	*0.78*	–0.08	*3*	2.2	73.0	75.2	0.87
FFPI-A agreeable	–0.25	–0.21	–0.14	0.02	0.09	*0.65*	–0.15	*2*	6.4	51.8	58.2	0.83
NEO-FFI-A agreeable	–0.30	–0.19	0.16	0.04	–0.07	*0.56*	*–0.41*	0	9.1	54.8	63.9	0.74
HPI-F-EMP empathetic	0.02	0.01	0.15	*0.33*	–0.03	*0.76*	–0.05	*2*	0.1	71.1	71.2	0.73
HPI-F-FRI friendly	0.01	0.00	*0.50*	0.17	0.13	*0.59*	–0.12	0	0.0	66.5	66.5	0.71
HPI-F-ROM romantic	0.24	0.00	*0.46*	*0.40*	0.10	*0.48*	–0.02	0	5.6	61.1	66.7	0.71
HPI-D-R risk seeking	0.00	–0.17	0.09	0.06	0.12	–0.01	*0.88*	*3*	0.0	82.6	82.6	0.88
HPI-F-TOR tough-reckless	0.27	–0.06	0.12	–0.06	0.04	–0.23	*0.78*	*3*	7.3	68.6	75.9	0.84
HPI-F-AMB ambitious	0.04	–0.13	0.01	–0.10	*0.40*	–0.01	*0.75*	*1*	0.1	75.4	75.5	0.75
HPI-F-HER heroic	0.18	–0.05	*0.37*	0.30	–0.07	–0.06	*0.73*	*1*	3.2	77.4	80.6	0.81
HPI-F-DOM charismatic	0.06	–0.13	*0.44*	0.05	0.13	–0.14	*0.71*	*1*	0.4	74.8	75.2	0.83
HPI-F-ADV adventurous	0.11	–0.05	0.04	*0.31*	–0.21	0.03	*0.70*	*2*	1.1	64.1	65.2	0.85
HPI-F-ENT enterprising	0.04	–0.12	*0.32*	0.10	*0.39*	–0.23	*0.64*	*1*	0.2	74.3	74.5	0.83
% explained all scales	17.9	8.6	11.4	6.8	7.9	6.9	13.0		17.9	54.6	72.5	0.84
% explained 12 DSM-IV	38.5	5.9	10.0	2.1	4.6	4.1	8.0		38.5	34.7	73.2	0.89
% explained 24 PD scales	38.5	7.4	5.8	3.8	4.2	4.1	8.8		38.5	34.1	72.6	0.88

MV stat. = marker variable status, see Methods; EV GDP = explained variance for the GDP factor; EV SFM = explained variance for the SFM (including R); EV 7 fac. = explained variance for GDP and SFM; CA = Cronbach's α (internal consistency), the last three values in this column are means for all 62 scales, for 12 DSM-IV PD scales and for 24 PD scales. All loadings above 0.30 are set in italics.

Variables

The study also intended to replicate the big five dimensions. The following three inventories were used to establish the FFM framework: the German NEO-FFI by Borkenau and Ostendorf [56], the German version of the FFPI by Hendricks et al. [57] and an experimental version of the Hamburg Personality Inventory (HPI-D) constructed by the author [48]. The FFPI is a modified big five inventory with a quite different variant of the fifth dimension, here called 'intellect/autonomy'. The HPI-D is based on a six-factor model (SFM), where BD-R is added to an only slightly modified FFM.

Additionally, 22 experimental facet scales (HPI-F) are explored in this study covering the whole range of the six basic factors. Three facets were devised for each of four FFM domains. BD-O obtained four facets because of its less well-replicated structure. For the BD-R domain, six facets were constructed to overcome the 'blind spot' the FFM seems to have in this trait area. This is a legitimate strategy in case of such deficiencies. A factor analytic study of Hoffmann, Andresen and Pawlik [unpubl. data] with four inventories (CPS, 16PF, NEO-FFI, HPI-D) showed that the sixth factor BD-R definitely could be replicated, but due to missing appropriate own facets was too much distorted by facets of other inventories that are rather peripheral to the BD-R construct.

Finally, the Inventory of Clinical Personality Accentuations (ICP) constructed by the author [58] was included. It comprises 18 scales, 12 of them strictly measuring the criterion-based contents of DSM-IV axis II disorders (ICP-G). The other six scales (ICP-E) cover further PD concepts, in part additionally or differently described by ICD-10. For instance, ICD-10 proposes an impulsive PD as a variant of the borderline PD. But also traditional German psychopathic personality concepts by Schneider [59] like the 'asthenic PD' were included. Further, six exploratory PD scales (ICP-P) were used like, for instance, the 'alexithymic', the 'harm avoidant and hypochondriacal' or the 'oppositional and reactant' PD.

Number of items per scale varied between 8 and 28, with the majority of scales having 12–24 items. The 18 ICP-G and -E scales uniformly have 18 items. These different scale lengths are the main source of different reliabilities reported in table 1. Some lower reliabilities also resulted from the explorative nature of six scales.

Statistical Methods

All scales used were analyzed for reliability, Cronbach's α (internal consistency) was calculated and documented for every scale. The Pearson correlations also were determined. Principal component factor analysis with subsequent orthogonal Varimax rotation was used.

Principal component analysis (PCA) was preferred because of its simple but exact mathematical logic. Of course, it is recognized that PCA does not safeguard against coextraction of limited amounts of error variance. This principally will lead to limited enhancements of percentages for explained reliable variance of scales compared with classical factor analysis based on communality estimates and iteration. But practically, in cases of applying conservative rules to the decision on the number of factors [60, 61], PCA renders almost identical factor results compared to classical common factor analysis. A critical analysis of PCA methodology is given by the author in the context of basic personality factor research [8].

Varimax rotation was chosen to have the possibility of descriptive variance fractionation. The sum of squared loadings can thus be split into additive contributions of the single factors. Of course, an orthogonal rotation does not exclude substantial correlations on the scale measurement level. Nevertheless, the possible correlational status of the factor-based scales can be approximately anticipated by inspection of the secondary loadings of the marker scales and by the correlational results well known for these established scales beyond the reported study.

The crucial decision on the number of factors was based on complex criteria including: eigenvalues greater than 1, minimum variance extraction for each scale, number of marker variables and, last but not least, considerations regarding factor replication. Five solutions (5–9 factors extracted and rotated) are analyzed in detail.

A marker variable criterion is used that was developed by the author [8]. This criterion discriminates three levels of a marker variable: level 1 is defined by a minimum dominant loading (abs.) of 0.45 and a minimum quotient of the dominant loading (abs.) to the highest secondary loading (abs.) of 1.5; level 2 is defined in analogue form with values of 0.60 and 2.0; level 3 uses values of 0.75 and 2.5.

Results

Principal Component Analysis

The PCA decomposition of the intercorrelation matrix resulted in nine eigenvalues greater than 1.0 (15.01, 11.37, 7.40, 5.28, 3.18, 1.76, 1.31, 1.18, 1.01). Due to the great number of scales and despite their high internal consistency level (table 1), it is not advisable to go beyond the Kaiser-Guttman rule of extraction. The decision concerning the adequate number of factors was also influenced by the goal of this study to test factors for substantial additional explanation of PD scale variance beyond the FFM (which, therefore, is needed as a standard structure for comparison).

A complete big five model was only achieved (as a subsystem) within the eight-factor solution (8-FS). In the 7-FS, BD-O was not existent as a separate factor, the respective NEO- and HPI-O domain scales loaded on BD-A and BD-R positively and on BD-C negatively. The extension to eight factors resulted in the expected BD-O the first time in the extraction process. In this FS, the expected sixth factor, BD-R, also showed up clearly together with a 'general dysfunctional personality' (GDP) factor and a minor 'autonomy' factor with very poor loading status. The latter had only substantial loadings greater than 0.30 for three scales (FFPI-IA, intellect-autonomy, 0.58, HPI-F-SES 0.49, IKP-G-DEP 0.44, all had also substantial loadings on other factors) and had only a sum of squared loadings of 1.61 compared with the range of 4.24–11.08 for the other rotated factors. The number of marker variable points (only 1) was also far below the fixed minimum of 4. The interpretability of this factor is also very questionable. It was decided to omit it in further documentation and consideration. As orthogonal Varimax rotation was used, where loadings represent exact correlations with the factors, this 'neglect' does not alter the loadings and variance contributions and fractionation of the other seven factors. Of course, this does not mean that rerotating the substantial seven factors with Varimax without the minor rotated eighth factor would result in exactly the same loading pattern. But the error would probably be small. Nevertheless, post hoc elimination of minor orthogonal factors bears a further risk of factor manipulation which is already massively given by the heterogenous rules for the primary decision of number of factors. This risk was accepted because comprehensiveness of description was the leading methodological principle in this study and in the model building of the author. Based on the experience with many data sets, in explorative factor analysis comprehensiveness very often implies an extraction routine just reaching the field where marginal noninterpretable factors appear after rotation. This legitimates a post hoc judgement of substantial and marginal or residual factors. These separations in many cases cannot be achieved by a prerotational reduction of extracted factors. In the reported study, a reduction to seven extracted components would miss BD-O which appears with full interpretability and three good marker variables in the rotated solution with eight factors.

A careful inspection regarding secondary loadings of the main BD-O scales in the Varimax 8-FS shows that in any case the separation of BD-O from the above-mentioned factors is warranted, and the potential intercorrelations on the scale level will be moderate, within the expectations set by the literature.

A check of the marker variable criteria used by the author in several studies [7] was selectively done for a comparison of the 8- and the 9-FSs. The latter was roughly equivalent in the total count of marker variable points, but failed to reach the minimum number of marker variable points for three factors. In the 9-FS again, the FFM was not fully replicated as a partial system because BD-A and BD-O collapsed into one broader factor and split off two minor factors with very poor loading status. So the 8-FS remained as the only convincing basis to answer the questions raised in this study. Thus, this factor analysis showed again that the decision on the number of factors in explorative factor analysis is crucial and complex and deserves critical attention and methodological scrutiny.

As to the 5-FS, a short note is also necessary. This pattern also showed no BD-O. It represents a dimensional reduction with no replication of the FFM. Here, the GDP factor did not yet show up, BD-N and BD-R are bloated and biased with many PD scales. It should be recognized that normal dimensions of personality may be empirically distorted if they are heavily loaded by PD scales in a factor analysis comprising the normal and clinical domains. Even if the normal FFM scales reach prominent loadings, an informational shift of factor meaning may take place, so that the loadings of clinical scales on these normal clinical hybrid factors can no longer be interpreted in terms of variance explained by the well-established normal basic factors. Therefore, factor analysis of normal and clinical scales often leads to ambiguous results, especially if underextraction far below the consistency level of the analyzed scales is practiced.

The new dimension BD-R is unequivocally present with approximately the same loading pattern from the 5-FS to all higher solutions up to nine factors. It is among the structurally very stable dimensions (BD-E, BD-C, BD-R), not much influenced by the decision on the number of factors, probably because of its rather elaborate underpinning with facet scales.

Table 1 presents the Varimax loading matrix for the seven substantial factors of the 8-FS. Several row and column sums of squared loading, expressed as percent of explained variance, are calculated. Additionally, the marker status of variables is given (see Method) and Cronbach's α consistencies documented to check whether this higher dimensional solution (compared to the big five) already explains the scales beyond the upper border defined by the internal consistency of the scales.

To begin with the latter point: the sums of squared loadings of all scales are below or just reach the consistency limit, thus the accepted seven factors may – with due caution because of the principal error contamination of PCA – be assumed to operate almost exclusively with 'true variance' according to the classical theory of testing.

Nearly all variables, the clinical scales included, are explained to a high degree above approximately three quarters of their reliable variance. Only five scales fall short of this margin, with three of them being above two thirds of reliable variance, the two weakest scales still being clearly above 50%.

General Dysfunctional Personality

The strongest factor with 10 marker variables – all DSM-IV or additional PD scales – is interpreted as a GDP factor. The highest loadings are given for PD syndromes that show some sort of cognitive aberration (delusional beliefs, perceptual distortions, dissociative aberrations of consciousness and mental functions, loss of cognitive control of affect, intrusions of unwanted thoughts and impulses, lack of mental recovery, sleep disturbances, ambivalent cognitions and emotions, disorganization of thought, behavior and affect). In fact, all PD scales loaded to a substantial but quite different degree on this GDP factor.

GDP explains 38.5% of the DSM-IV variance and also of the extended set of 24 PDs. The six normal dimensions of the solution including the RC factor predict less variance (34.7% for DSM-IV PDs; 34.1% for all PDs). The FFM alone explains only 26.7% for DSM-IV PDs and 25.3% for all PDs.The latter percentages roughly correspond with the mean multiple correlation predictions (about 0.30) obtained in the literature for pure questionnaire studies.

Neuroticism

Neuroticism/emotional lability shows quite strong loading overlap with the GDP factor. The neuroticism scales of all three FFM/SFM inventories show also loadings about 0.50 on GDP. Only two facets focussing on emotional lability show a marker status. This loading overlap leads to a correlation of about 0.50 between GDP and BD-N on the scale measurement level. It would be an illusion to believe that it could be possible to perfectly orthogonalize these two factorial constructs. The 'negative affect' center of BD-N will always lead to a moderate but substantial correlation. Of course, this does not mean that it would be unwise to 'normalize' BD-N as much as possible. The existence of a truly abnormal GDP factor favors the option to reinterpret and restructure neuroticism as 'quite normal' sensitiveness, emotional lability and disposition for negative affect.

In this context, it is interesting to note that the loadings of PD scales on BD-N are not as prominent as expected. The leading syndrome on this factor is the hypothetical stress-prone PD flanked by secondary loadings of depressive, asthenic, explosive and borderline PD scales. The percentage of DSM-IV variance explained by BD-N is only 5.9%, and for all 24 PD scales it goes up to 7.4%. In this respect, BD-N is no longer leading among the six basic normal factors. BD-R shows higher values (DSM-IV PDs 8.0%; all PDs 8.8%). But the PD scale loadings on BD-N are generally positive with almost no exception. BD-R, however, gives strong positive and negative correlational contributions to PDs. With this unidirectional loading pattern for PD scales, BD-N still seems to be unique among the six normal dimensions found here. Possibly BD-N has some unique properties in this study because the main loadings are given for scales focussing on 'stability', the negative pole of BD-N. Therefore, the comparatively very low level of PD prediction should be regarded with due caution.

Extraversion

Dimension BD-E shows a clear structure with no surprising results, but it should be noted that this broad dimension includes dominant and submissive, assertive and warm qualities [62]. There exist variants of BD-E in the literature, especially based on the Goldberg adjectival instruments [63] which are strongly biased towards 'boldness' and other contents of BD-R. Such hybrid dominance/assertiveness/surgency BD-E/BD-R dimensions represent a minority position, but it has led to the widespread opinion that BD-R is a subcomponent of BD-E. This definitely is not true, as can be easily derived from this study. Nevertheless, it is also very clear that the discrimination between BD-R and BD-E may become difficult if a strongly biased sample of facets is constructed or chosen. One major consideration to achieve this separation is the focus on positive affect, optimism, liveliness and cheerful gregariousness for measurement of BD-E.

BD-E shows a strong factorial explanation of DSM-IV PD scales, namely the schizoid, avoidant and depressive syndromes at the negative pole and the histrionic syndrome at the positive pole. A hyperthymic/hypomanic PD which, unfortunately, was not represented in our scale repertoire would obviously also load on the positive pole of BD-E.

Openness to Experience

Dimension BD-O, as mentioned before, had some problems to be separated from BD-A, BD-R and BD-C(–). This may have to do with the weaker scale basis. The FFPI-IA scale is no marker variable of BD-O and scatters its loadings over several factors including the marginal eighth factor. This implies that the FFPI is no complete big five inventory in the sense of the mainstream consensus following the model of Costa and McCrae [64]. Furthermore, three of the four proposed marker facets of BD-O load higher on BD-R or BD-E.

Of special interest is the loading pattern of the intelligence scale that loads dominantly on BD-R and also shows substantial positive loadings on BD-C and BD-O. This scale describes a gifted, intelligent person with high mental efficiency regardless of cognitive style (best item: 'I am very intelligent'). It is well known that such self-report scales for the 'g factor of intelligence' are only poor in their correlation with test intelligence [65]. It therefore can preferentially be seen as an affirmatively expressed motivation to possess and excel high 'mental power' in the context of competition seeking. The dominant but moderate loading (0.48) on BD-R seems plausible in this context. As a side effect of this result, it no longer seems adequate to interpret and name BD-O as 'intellect'. BD-O and BD-C obviously both integrate certain opposing cognitive styles. Accordingly, the weaker and rather unstable basis of the 'true' BD-O factor can be traced back to conceptual problems and misconceptions of this construct at the border to the intelligence domain. In the opinion of the author, BD-O has lost its global affinity to intelligence, and even the small but replicated correlation with measured intelligence could be interpreted as an artifact of a cognitive style bias in test intelligence measures [48].

As to PD scale loadings, BD-O is rather poor for DSM-IV constructs, but if new concepts like, for instance, the alexithymic or regressive personalities are included, its PD relevance will increase. As Widiger and Costa noted [1], the poor PD explanation of BD-O is probably only limited to the clinical personality syndromes favored today. Maladaptive personality traits in strong affinity to the negative and positive poles of BD-O can also be found in the history of PD description (e.g. 'pseudologia phantastica') proposed by Schneider [59].

Conscientiousness

Conscientiousness is well marked with the three domain scales of the established inventories. Interestingly, the conservatism scale is highly correlated with BD-C and a little lower with BD-O(–). This is in good agreement with the proposal of the author [66] – see also Riemann et al. [67] – that BD-O and BD-C define and predict together the concept of conservatism originally defined psychometrically by Wilson and Patterson [68]. Other authors come to the conclusion that only BD-O should be considered relevant for this main dimension of conservative (vs. liberal or radical) attitudes [69]. Taking several studies together, an equal relevance of the cognitive style dimensions BD-O *and* BD-C for the main conservative-progressive axis of attitudes can be assumed. This is especially clear for conceptions of BD-C close to rigidity [70].

The prediction of DSM-IV PD scales is poor for BD-C and limited to the compulsive syndrome. If all 24 PD scales are considered, BD-C is comparable to BD-O in general explanatory potency. Both cognitive dimensions belong to the low PD prediction group of basic factors in the NEOCAR system. This may change if more attitudinally defined PDs would be accepted (e.g. authoritarian PD).

Agreeableness

Agreeableness is optimally marked by the HPI-D-A scale which focusses on altruistic behavior, nurturance, tenderness, charity and striving for peaceful harmony. The FFM trait of BD-A is somewhat less relevant. Aggression and antagonism are also less present at the negative pole. Therefore the loadings of FFPI- and NEO-FFI-A are lower and in the case of NEO-A also scattered. The latter loads also negatively on BD-R (–0.41) and GDP (–0.30). For the BD-A construct, a trend towards lower statistical and content homogenity is evident, especially for NEO-A scales, as shown, for instance, by Hoffmann, Andresen and Pawlik [unpubl. data].

The PD prediction of BD-A in this solution is remarkably low for DSM-IV and the extended PDs (only the antisocial PD shows a substantial negative loading), quite contrary to the literature on FFM-A. The content shift away from the NEO-A scale may be most relevant for this effect. But it can be assumed that another sampling of PD concepts could enhance the predictive potency. The positive pole of BD-A does not have a substantial loading from any PD. This could change if sensitively empathetic, hypersentimental, dysfunctionally tender-hearted or self-defeating traits would be included. On the other pole, sadistic PD would strengthen the clinical impact of BD-A. Of course, the definition of PDs in the direction of prosocial traits is inhibited by the traditional definition of psychopathy which stresses the aggressive or anti-/asocial qualities of PD.

Risk and Competition Seeking

Finally, BD-R is well replicated in this study. The only domain scale of the HPI-D reaches a pure high marker status, and the six facet scales also are marker variables. The facets show several secondary loadings on BD-E, BD-O and BD-C, but not on BD-N and BD-A. Therefore, the idea that BD-R and BD-A are separated artificially is far away from reality. Test construction led to quite orthogonal scales [48]. From the viewpoint of opponent dynamic traits (as elaborated in the discussion) 'tough' and 'tender' traits may go together in one individual. 'Risking/fighting' and 'caring/helping' are no contradiction, but strong contrast traits with possible synergistic function, as, for instance, displayed in 'civilian courage', where strong social motives go together with risk taking.

BD-R is loaded by anxious-fearful and harm-avoidant PDs on one side and antisocial, aggressive, oppositional and narcissistic maladaptivity on the other side. Surprisingly, BD-R is a rather strong incremental factor for the total PD explanation beyond the FFM with approximately 10% of the reliably PD scale variance.

Multiple Explanations

The seven-factor model including the factor GDP reaches an explanation of about 73% of total PD scale variance of DSM-IV and in the extended 24 PD scale system. If the consistency values of single PD scales are taken into account, the explanatory power amounts to about 80% of true variance. For all practical purposes (e.g. screening diagnosis), this is a sufficient level. This statement is also justified as the span of explained variance for single PD scales is tolerable (53–82%, uncorrected), and the outlier reduction for the dependent PD (53%, next lowest value is 63%) may be explained by special aspects of the ICP dependency scale limiting their PD relevance. The appropriate interpretation is that seven dimensions are sufficient to explain all PD scales within an integrative model.

The predictive power of the GDP factor is higher than the combined effect of the six normal dimensions (38.5 vs. 34.5%). This also is quite independent of a narrow or extended sample of PD scales. But here, the relative factor sources of single PDs are quite different. Some PD scales are mainly explained by GDP, others show a much higher influence of normal dimensions. It is assumed that this is an aspect of the severity of the PD item content. But other rivaling explanations are possible.

Discussion

The study presented here began with a critical evaluation of the FFM of normal personality contradicting its claim to also account for all PDs. A literature survey showed that the empirical evidence does not substantiate this hypothesis. The PD comprehensiveness of the FFM only amounted to about 50% of the supposedly reliable PD questionnaire variance. Several options and ideas to enhance this modest explanatory power were considered, but no definite conclusion could be reached on the grounds of the existing literature.

An empirical study was therefore conducted aiming at an integrative model to explain representative normal and clinical personality scales in one comprehensive dimensional system. Six normal factors were replicated including a slightly modified FFM and a sixth basic factor, BD-R, postulated by the author [7]. Additionally, a broad psychopathological factor called GDP was found that shows some loading overlap and a scale-based correlation of about 0.50 with BD-N. The other six factors are virtually orthogonal (in the correlational range of ±0.30 for scales constructed on the basis of the factors).

Whereas the FFM part of the factor solution would alone only explain 25% of the PD scale variance, the seven-factor solution including the broad GDP dimension accounts for 73%. This can be interpreted as full PD comprehensiveness if internal consistencies are taken into account.

The conclusion is reached that the FFM (1) definitely has to be extended by the sixth orthogonal factor BD-R and (2) can – after the incorporation of BD-R – be most economically complemented by a seventh factor of GDP to account for all undisputable PD scales. This GDP factor shows especially high loadings of cognitively aberrant PDs.

It should be added that an ongoing study of the author with a much larger sample of scales (295 from 14 inventories) yielded a similar GDP factor with slight modifications [unpubl. data]. Here, GDP accounted for a lower proportion of PD variance. BD-N was more massively loaded by subaffective and neurotic PD syndromes, so that BD-N gains a higher predictive power for PD scales – in contrast to the study reported here where BD-N is surprisingly normal in this respect. Therefore, a definite and stable consensus regarding the percentages of PD prediction for a new standard set of basic factors definitely needs further empirical studies combining factor analytic, test operational and regression analytic approaches based on very large samples of scales and subjects.

The Sixth Normal Factor: BD-R

The author postulates a sixth basic factor (BD-R) [7, 66] based on ten own large-scale factor analytic questionnaire studies [8, 9, 71, 72] and several works of other researchers [73–75]. This factor again is fully replicated in this eleventh study with a convincing status as a broadly defined, basically orthogonal factor, quite comparable to the equally replicated factors of the FFM.

BD-R in this study is well marked by six facet scales with loadings above 0.60. The domain BD-R scale of the HPI-D is clearly the best marker variable with very good simple structure, a high loading of 0.88 and no secondary loading above 0.17. It seems important to note that HPI-D-R has a loading on BD-A of –0.01, and HPI-D-A has a loading on BD-R of –0.08. As HPI-D-R and HPI-D-A have communalities of 0.83 and 0.75 (with internal consistencies of 0.88 and 0.87), it can be concluded that BD-R and BD-A have an upper limit of –0.30 on the scale correlation level. This low correlation level was replicated for the final scales of the HPI [48] in several independent data sets. This latter point has to be stressed because NEO-FFI-A loads on both BD-R (–0.41) and BD-A (0.56) which might suggest that the factors BD-R and BD-A found here are highly correlated subfactors of an underlying bipolar antagonism-agreeableness factor optimally marked by NEO-FFI-A. This is not the case. BD-R and BD-A are as *approximately* independent of each other as BD-N and BD-E or BD-C and BD-O.

BD-R adds substantial PD scale variance explanation (about 10%), surprisingly more than any other normal basic factor. These contributions are mainly relevant for harm avoidance, fearfulness and phobic avoidance PD scales, but only in the domain of physical and environmental threat and risk, not substantially for social fears. On the other hand, substantial contributions are given for the antisocial, narcissistic and sadistic PD scales, also including maladaptive oppositional, aggressive and risk-accentuated sensation-seeking traits.

As can be seen from the loading pattern of facets, BD-R is not a narrow trait of more or less maladaptive risk taking [76–78] bloated artificially to become a pseudo second-order factor. Several important traits come together to define this new basic dimension, currently called BD-R. The title may be preliminary and too narrow, as most short titles are; therefore a broader description must be given here.

BD-R+, for instance, means traits like adventurousness and preference for dangerous outdoor activities, extreme sports and forceful physical acting out. Enterprising activities and risk achievement in economical and business contexts, competitive and assertive attitudes and behaviors in diverse fields of rivalry, leadership ambitions, and career also belong to the spectrum, but show some overlap with factor BD-C. BD-R+ personalities like challenges, they have a 'strong ego', motivation to win competitions and master dangerous situations leading to all sorts of active longing, fighting and risking. Technical interests and strivings for handycraft or engineering competence are also aspects of BD-R+. BD-R+ persons sometimes become 'heroes' and powerful leaders, but they also can live marginal solitary lives, for instance, as 'trappers' or 'survival freaks'.

The concept of risk preference is also a basic aspect of the sensation-seeking construct proposed by Zuckerman [79]. But it has been shown by the author [80] that only the subscale 'thrill and adventure seeking' in the classical sensation-seeking scale (SSS-V) by Zuckerman et al. [81] belongs to the basic factor BD-R, whereas, for instance, SSS-V 'experience seeking' is a marker variable for BD-O. The large-scale factor analysis mentioned above makes it very clear that the basic factor scale of the ZKPQ (impulsive unsocialized sensation seeking) claimed by Zuckerman et al. [82] to be a superior alternative to the factor BD-O has a multiple loading pattern on several factors and does not constitute or mark clearly one of the well-established basic factors. Nevertheless, a negative loading dominance on BD-C can be seen, as also reported by Zuckerman et al. [83] later on. This state of affairs makes the many psychobiological findings [84] gathered with the classical SSS-V (or the ZKPQ) very hard to integrate into the basic factor model and especially the factor BD-R presented here.

The whole 'facet landscape' of BD-R is currently explored in the large-scale study mentioned above [unpubl. data]. It is quite possible that BD-R will prove to be even broader than expected, for instance, with regard to the excessive use of new media. Exploration of the lower hierarchical levels of this basic personality dimension has just begun.

The Factor GDP: Its Meaning and Problems

A factor of GDP has already been – in quite different terminology – a topic in FFM research. Replicating Tellegen [85] – see also Benet and Waller [46] – Saucier and Goldberg [86] evaluated a factor of 'negative valence' or 'low base rate attributes' as definitely being 'beyond the big five'. But this traditional adjective-bound personality research is far away from a thorough clinical evaluation of this additional 'negative self' factor. Furthermore, the phenomenological breadth of this factor seems to be underestimated in adjectival 'beyond FFM' research. The predominant interpretations are directed at response styles and artificial influences due to inadequate proband behavior, e.g. random responding [86]. These are legitimate but very restricted concerns. In fact, the mainstream of differential psychology did not find a convincing and constructive answer to the intriguing nature of this construct. Correlational comparisons with PD scales have not been reported.

GDP and the Definition of PD Psychopathology. The GDP dimension added to the 'basic six' forming only one broad 'plural' PD component seems to capture the definitely psychopathological variance of all PD scales. One quite plausible extension of this assumption would be that the loadings of single PD scales on the six normal dimensions per se represent normal variance. This concept stands in sharp contrast to Widiger [87] who stated:

> 'To the extent that maladaptive personality traits are extreme variants of normal personality traits (...), the degree of deviation on any particular NEO-PI-R domain or facet scale would suggest maladaptivity. For the most part, this will, in fact, be the case (...)' [87, pp 313–314].

Thus, in the SFM + GDP model of our study, some of the 24 PD scales could be categorized as less psychopathological (like, for instance, the depressive, oppositional, labile, schizoid, avoidant, histrionic, antisocial, fearful, narcissistic or compulsive PDs) because they are more explained by the six normal dimensions compared to GDP.

Other PD scales (schizotypal, obsessiotypal, negativistic, anxious, dissociative, asthenic, paranoid and borderline) may belong to the severer forms which show more explanation by the GDP factor. This would be principally concordant with different levels of severity postulated for different PDs in the literature [88]. Nevertheless, caution is indicated, because psychopathologic severity derived from loading pattern may be heavily influenced by item content and style beyond the target criteria. For instance, narcissism items may be formulated as very pathological, but also closer to normality, and this principally applies to all PD concepts. Of course, this does not exclude the possibility that different criteria sets of PD are genuinely – rather independent of item writing style – closer to normality, like, for instance, the histrionic and obsessive-compulsive PDs [88].

GDP may be influenced by social desirability or inconsistency/infrequency response styles. In this study, no check could be made regarding such constructs. Preliminary evidence [58] makes infrequency responding somewhat more probable as a possible serious contamination. Social desirability is a greater problem for BD-N scales. The inconsistency problem appears unsolved yet, because alogical/irrational/erratic responding may in part be a symptom of severe generalized PD, and in particular schizotypal personality.

GDP and Axis I–Axis II Comorbidity. In our study, it could not be definitely excluded that axis I symptomatology enters into the data. Of course, the instruction, of the questionnaires ask more or less intensely and efficiently for the normal and usual way of experiencing and behaving. Episodic phenomena and unusual short-lived moments of crisis should not enter into the self-description of traits. But definite evidence is missing on whether this rule was followed by the participants. This critical point remains to be evaluated in future studies, where valid axis I screening instruments should also be included as covariates. This would be an unusually high effort in research on basic factors with a large number of volunteers. But to put the hypothesis of a GDP factor – definitely positioned on axis II – to a crucial test, such a scrupulous differential diagnosis is indispensable, mainly because substantial comorbidity between axis I and axis II syndromes is well known [89, 90].

General PD Criteria and Internal PD Comorbidity. It should also be considered that the GDP factor may simply represent central aspects of the *overarching* definition of PDs that are bound to the general PD criteria of DSM-IV [22]. And these common generalizing features of all PDs, regardless of their different psychosocial makeups, may also be the main reason for the high level of internal PD comorbidity which is evident in thorough diagnostic studies using standard interview techniques [91]. These studies came to the conclusion that – if a PD diagnosis is definite – this is mostly a plural diagnosis (with a mean of about four coprevalent single PDs in the cited study). Such studies also show that a GDP factor with high internal PD comorbidity as its logical diagnostical consequence cannot be a matter of questionnaire methods. It seems to be a genuine phenomenon [92].

GDP and Psychosis Proneness. Could GDP be interpreted as a general factor of psychosis proneness? At first glance, this might seem plausible, but closer inspection of the PD scale contributions makes it clear that this interpretation would seem at least premature. Several scales that are quite different from the contents of psychosis proneness scales contribute as marker variables to the reported study. Therefore, the interpretation is preliminarily favored that GDP cuts across traditional spectrum concepts of psychosis proneness and neurosis proneness. The core attribute of high GDP is its assumed psychopathological severity with strong dyscognitive elements of various forms. This aberration may appear obsessive (as a classical neurotic form with strong resistance), schizotypal or paranoid (with strong delusional aspects in terms of psychosis proneness), or emotionally dysregulated or dyscontrolled (as an affective or borderline disorder). All these spectrum aspects, and some more, are incorporated into this GDP factor. Tradition-bound diagnostically guided research may have some problems to accept such a conglomerate factor, although its empirical status is quite strong in this study.

Nevertheless, the new large-scale study mentioned above gives somewhat more evidence in favor of the psychosis proneness interpretation. A final decision should be based on further studies including special instruments and psychobiological paradigms, as developed particularly in research on schizotypy [54].

A Hypothetical Three-System Model for the SFM and some Implications for Psychobiological Research on Basic Normal Dimensions

The structural theory of basic factors presented by the author [7–9, 48] gained its initial impetus through the emergence of the sixth basic factor BD-R. This enabled a perspective on three hypothetical systems of factor pairs, which operate in a well-demarcated subfield of personal functioning and may have an antagonistic/synergistic relation. It must be conceded that the underlying nature of this postulated relation between pairs of factors in the same domain of traits remains hypothetical and also somewhat vague empirically. Of course, it also handles with dynamic psychobiological ideas, where rather static correlational data are the prime sources of structures. Nevertheless, this basic idea seems promising for future research. The descriptive and heuristic value of the 'three-pair approach' remains substantial if the notion of opponent psychobiological dynamism behind these dual basic traits is not yet accepted as explicative and verified.

System I – Temperament, Affect and Mood. This subsystem is formed by the core temperamental factors BD-N and BD-E, both mainly defined by their affective and mood qualities in the context of social behavior and emotional relationships. Therefore, these two factors are also described as positive affect and negative affect [93]. They probably are so highly interwoven biopsychosocially [72] that separate research on one of the two complementing factors seems very risky. Together, mainly this pair of factors regulates general well-being, optimism-pessimism, habitual mood and life satisfaction [94]. Decades ago, finding this approximate orthogonality of contradictive traits was a great surprise [95], today it is basic knowledge. This should be kept in mind when the same basic principle is postulated for the other two factor pairs (subsystems).

BD-N and BD-E have been the main focus of multivariate psychophysiological personality research [72, 96] and biological theory building [97–99]. This field of personality studies is heavily influenced by general research on the biopsychology of stress, activation and emotional reactions [100] and from the very beginning has been flanked by differential psychopharmacology [97, 101].

System II – Cognition, Values and Attitudes. System II comprises BD-O and BD-C. Up to now, the opposite properties of these two cognitive factors have not been fully recognized. Both factors have an affinity to contrasting attitudinal orientation, especially regarding the well-known general factor radicalism-conservatism. Religious orientation and moral value systems are similarly polarized. BD-C+ scorers tend towards orthodox clerical and moralistic orientation, BD-O+ scorers typically favor a liberal esoteric-spiritual and humanistic orientation. Likewise, BD-C+ and BD-O+ persons have contrasting cognitive styles, thinking and working habits (convergent-normative vs. divergent-alternative). Life-styles and esthetic preferences are also pseudocontradictory (conformistic vs. unconventional, traditional vs. modern). Regarding affective and phantasy processes, BD-C+ tends towards control and repression, BD-O+ towards accentuation/sensibilization and regression. As with BD-N and BD-E, it must be stressed that the correlation of BD-O and BD-C is negative, but very low. Therefore, their contrasting description does not exclude that one individual has high scores on both styles, thinking habits or beliefs. Here also both factors constitute a balanced interwoven system. It does not seem useful to separate them in whatever validation context.

As to psychobiological research, no 'mainstream' has to be commented, because this pair of basic factors surprisingly has not attracted much biological interest, especially not as a subsystem. This is even true for cognitive neuropsychophysiology and neuropsychology, where potentially interesting hypotheses, like hemispheric differentiation/asymmetry and interhemispheric functional organization [102, 103], are definitely waiting to be linked hypothetically to this basic trait system which seems to determine our *'Weltanschauung'*, how 'we see and interpret the world'. Of course, research on the differential mental functions and 'cognitive styles' of the cortical hemispheres is very elaborated and allows many *indirect* associations with system II. But *directly*, the BD-O and BD-C scales of personality inventories have very rarely been the target of neuropsychobiological hypothesis testing in this field.

System III – Survival-Related Competitive/Risking and Cooperative/Protective Behavior. BD-R and a nurturant/helping BD-A, as reported in this study, are also much less founded psychobiologically, compared to BD-N and BD-E. They can be conceptualized as contrasting factors of (partly gender-related) habitual social roles along the main axis of tough and tender behavioral styles. Courageous and helping behaviors share some core elements of character traits, that is, of motivational traits ultimately relevant for the skilled and responsible mastery of danger, threat and other vital and existential challenges to oneself and other members of the community. Of course, BD-C and BD-O also comprise some (more cognition-based) elements of character and value orientation [62], but in system III forms of ego-/superego involvement with primary behavioral relevance deeply rooted in positively attributed archaic roles and 'archetypes' (e.g. 'hero', 'helper') seem to dominate. This factor pair probably has developed originally from primitive directly 'survival-related' behavioral systems and seems to incorporate gender roles to certain degrees. In evolutionary psychology 'competition' and 'cooperation' as separate complexes of motives and interactional styles which form a subtle system of balances have gained the status of a potent and popular explanatory paradigm [104], especially for behavior in conflict situations. But not only competitive and cooperative role taking is explained by BD-R and BD-A. Risk and competition seeking in particular goes beyond social roles and includes exploration, experimentation and challenge seeking in broadly expanded environmental (natural, technical) fields.

BD-R and BD-A are strongly contrasting in contents and connotations (tough vs. tender, cool vs. warm) but show an only weak negative correlation if factorial scales are constructed [48]. Between these two main motivation factors very important balancing and counterregulatory functions can be assumed, e.g. well-known in the context of aggression inhibition, where BD-R activity (fighting, challenging, aggression) shifts to BD-A activity (protecting, helping) when certain signals of submission are presented to the superior.

Psychobiological research is only poorly developed for BD-R and BD-A on the level of personality domain factors, especially not in combination of both [105]. The loosely associated gender roles have attracted somewhat

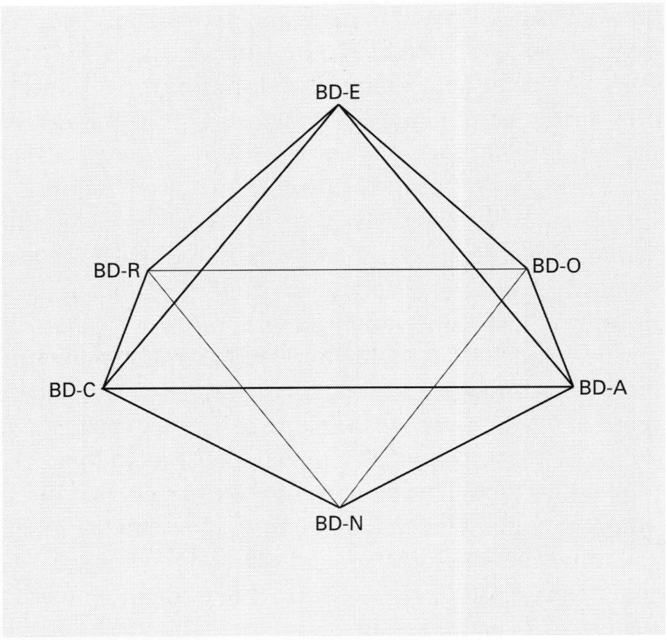

Fig. 1. Six basic personality dimensions as a regular octaeder distance model with three subsystems of opponent factors.

more interest among biologically oriented researchers, but simple relationships are not to be expected here, as revealed by the pioneering psycho- and biometric study of Netter-Munkelt [106]. Nevertheless, research on sexual hormones and related biological variables potentially seems to be very successful or promising in this field of behavior [107].

Clinically, BD-R and BD-A are correlated/loaded with tendencies towards antisocial and sadistic as well as fearful/phobic and self-defeating personality and empathetic disturbances. These syndromes are also substantially correlated with gender [58]. It can be concluded that the emergence of BD-R as a basic factor of personality offers a new 'two-factor' psychobiological paradigm for gender-related normal traits and associated clinical syndromes. This also means that the main theoretical concern of personality research should reintegrate those aspects of behavior, motives and interests that for a long time have been isolated in research on gender roles or sex differences [108].

The Geometric Model. Based on the synoptic evidence regarding factor and especially scale correlations from several own factor analytic and test construction studies [7, 8] targeting the six factors and their measurement, a hypothetical geometrical model was developed incorporating the three subsystems of slightly negatively correlated factor pairs. The mathematical aspects of the model are only approximately specified. The basic idea is to transform the intercorrelations of the six factors/scales into a distance function (positive correlations = shorter distance, negative correlations = longer distance) and to construct a three-dimensional form that approximates the resulting distance values. Of course, six-dimensional units cannot accurately be projected into a three-dimensional distance space, but in our case a quite satisfying approximation seems to be achieved synoptically. Figure 1 shows this structure in geometrically idealized form. A regular octaeder is the result, each factor being represented by an angle of the octaeder. It should be stressed that this geometrical representation should not be misunderstood as a classical geometrical factor plot. The logic behind is quite different. Synoptically derived from many empirical studies, the geometrical form chosen here has the following correlational basis: (1) the three factor pairs in each subsystem are characterized by weak negative correlations of about –0.30; (2) all other factor combinations show weak positive correlations around 0.10.

The utility of this model for more complex relationships will be demonstrated below, where connections with six hypothetical PD factors are postulated. Some correlations between FFM factors in the literature, for instance, the negative correlation of BD-C and BD-N based on the NEO-PI-R [64], seem to contradict this model. But the own HPI construction with BD-R as an additional construct leads to limited redefinitions and rotations of the other factors too. BD-C now is more defined by rigid behavior and thinking as also realized in other basic factor inventories [70], and these elements lead to a reapproachment of BD-N and BD-C.

It should be noted, as an experience from many test construction studies, that the six model dimensions can – within the narrow boundaries of about ± 0.30 – be 'shaped' by skilled test construction to fulfill certain correlational expectations. Therefore, it must be admitted that the definition of 'opponent pairs' of factors should not be solely based on such marginal and somewhat shaky statistical relations. Content and criterion validity aspects are more relevant and reliable, and they had much more influence on the emergence of the model than the patterns of factor intercorrelations in the framework of approximate orthogonality.

Can GDP Be 'Unfolded' into Replicable Subfactors and Does a Potential Oblique Six-Dimensional PD Model Show a Homologous Structure to the Basic Six Model?

If only PD scales are subjected to factor analysis, usually more than one factor, actually three or four, are obtained [37, 41–43]. They are more or less oblique, but a good differential interpretation based on definite marker variables is possible. Several authors presented much higher factor numbers on the item level. But the second-order analyses of these highly intercorrelated factorial syndromes again show the typical three or four factors [109].

Basically, the empirically derived position of the FFM is that PDs form factors roughly equivalent to the big five excluding BD-O [42, 43], and that in studies with normal and clinical scales these clinical dimensions fall together with the respective normal dimensions [26, 109].

The position presented here is that six dimensions for PD scales should arise if adequate representative sampling of syndromes, also going beyond DSM-IV and ICD-10, is achieved. The scale alexithymic PD in our study has already shown through its leading negative correlation with BD-O [1] that the latter is not a construct 'too far away from PDs'. This impression is obviously only the effect of unrepresentative PD diagnoses and scale selection. Following these lines of extended variable sampling, a first factor analysis of 324 ICP items clearly resulted in a statistically convincing oblique factor solution coming close to the own hypothesis [58].

The notion of six pathological dimensions is presented as an extension of the model of normal personality dimensions (fig. 2). Here, pathological dimensions constitute a more compact (short distance = oblique) but geometrically proportional structure compared to the virtually orthogonal model of normal personality.

The fact that clinical factors are more highly correlated, and that most PD scales are substantially and positively correlated with BD-N [110] is incorporated into the distance relations of the dual model. GDP is only an abstract element in this graphical representation defined by the first second-order component of six substantially correlated subfactors. The clinical dimensions are given equal abbreviations with the suffix 'd' added (for disordered).

First of all, this graphical model is not suggesting an empirical twelve-dimensional system – six normal *and* six abnormal. Such a system has never been demonstrated by factor analysis on the scale level. It should also be stressed that these six oblique clinical dimensions are only reliably

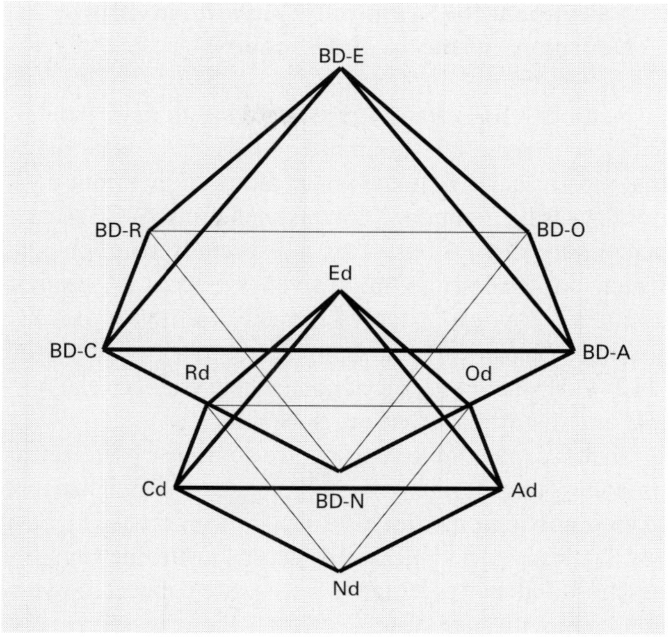

Fig. 2. Hypothetical dimensional structure of PD homologous to the basic six distance model. d = Disordered.

obtained if truly representative PD scale samples are analyzed without normal personality scales added. Nevertheless, splitting up GDP always means that contributions of the SFM are implicitly involved. The clinical SFM is in parts imported from the normal domains which are statistically combined with the powerful GDP influence to constitute the clinical six. Therefore, the seven-factor system including GDP and the dual normal versus abnormal SFM are no contradiction. They complement each other.

It must also be noted that the postulated six PD dimensions cannot be simple psychopathological variants of the normal SFM in terms of a one-to-one relation. The clinical PD factors will appear more unipolar than the more or less bipolar normal factors. This follows from first empirical evidence and algebraic considerations which cannot be discussed in detail here. These finer aspects of the hypothetical configuration of dimensional syndromes of the clinical SFM are presented elsewhere [58]. At the moment, the geometric-symbolic model of figure 2 must still be understood as a fascinating but also demanding and difficult hypothesis which can only be tackled successfully if several problems (for instance, representativeness of the included PDs) can be solved.

A Proposal for Systematic Advancements in Neuropsychobiological Research

Neuropsychobiological research relies in many studies [111] on diverse questionnaire constructs of personality that mostly lack a well-known, let alone an invariant positioning within a standard dimensional framework of basic personality dimensions. This is especially true for constructs and scales like 'impulsiveness', 'type A', 'aggressiveness', 'shyness', 'depressiveness', 'sensation/novelty seeking', 'harm avoidance/anxiety' or 'psychoticism' [112–114] which are placed somewhere between the normal and disturbed spheres of personality.

Such 'borderland' constructs are obviously preferred as predictors or criteria in psychobiological research because of their apparent medical and social relevance [115]. Several diathesis and vulnerability claims regarding somatic, psychosomatic or psychiatric disease are connected hypothetically with high (risk) scores on the respective questionnaire scales. The cumulative experience with this research practice using divergently expanding and differentiated questionnaire criteria is mainly negative because of numerous failures to replicate and systematize initially positive single findings based on special questionnaire scales [96, 116]. Of course, the reasons for the altogether poor empirical status of questionnaire-based psychobiological personality research also reach far beyond personality scale selection and construction. But these more basic problems cannot be thoroughly analyzed and overcome if the erratic influences of the questionnaire criteria remain as influential as it appears today.

According to the results and model presented, scales of whatever origin and purpose could be 'anchored' within an extended, truly comprehensive basic factor system beyond the incomprehensive big five and a characteristic combination of predictive weights could be determined that allows a matching with other scales without direct comparison. One of the main advantages of this model is the systematic distinction and dimensional construct explication of normal and disordered (maladaptive) personality dimensions.

As an example: the new personality system can possibly explain some disturbing discrepancies between various genetic studies of normal and clinical personality scales. Recently, a consensus has emerged that normal dimensions of personality are rather uniformly characterized by a substantial genetic contribution of about 50%, virtually no shared environmental (family) influence and a strong influence of individual nonshared environment [93, 117]. But there seem to be some exceptions to this rule. Bergeman et al. [118] reported results where NEO-PI-A shows much lower heritability than expected. This may be explained by the fact that according to our model and results NEO-FFI-A is 'hybrid' in its factorial composition within the SFM (and therefore rather inconsistent psychometrically) and additionally includes psychopathological variance (derived by its loading on GDP). For the latter dimension, the robust rule of thumb mentioned above regarding genetic and different environmental sources cannot be applied with sufficient safety. There are several researchers who consider that PD scales are less or inconsistently influenced by genetic factors and that other sources, also including shared family environment or traumata have to be taken into account [119–124]. A direct heritability test for the GDP factor has not yet been undertaken. A large-scale twin study should be started for the final HPI scales and their revision [48] including GDP and its highly oblique subsyndromes measured by the ICP [58].

Acknowledgments

I have to thank Steffen Moritz, and a competent reviewer for valuable comments on a first draft of this article. Many thanks also to Andrea Andresen who corrected the English text.

References

1 Widiger TA, Costa PT: Personality and personality disorders. J Abnorm Psychol 1994;103:78–91.
2 McCrae RR, John OP: An introduction to the Five-Factor Model and its applications. J Pers 1992;60:175–215.
3 Costa PT, McCrae RR: Domains and facets: Hierarchical personality assessment using the revised NEO Personality Inventory. J Pers Assess 1995;64:21–50.
4 Brand CR: Open to experience – Closed to intelligence: Why the 'Big Five' are really the 'Comprehensive Six'. Eur J Pers 1994;8:299–310.
5 Block J: A contrarian view of the five-factor approach to personality description. Psychol Bull 1995;117:187–215.
6 Becker P: Wie big sind die Big Five? (How big are the Big Five?). Z Diff Diagn Psychol 1996;17:209–221.
7 Andresen B: Risikobereitschaft (R) – Der sechste Basisfaktor der Persönlichkeit: Konvergenz multivariater Studien und Konstruktexplikation (Risk preference (R) – The sixth basic factor of personality: Convergence of multivariate studies and construct explication). Z Diff Diagn Psychol 1995;16:210–236.
8 Andresen B: Persönlichkeitsstruktur und Psychosetendenz (Personality Structure and Psychotic Tendency). Westerau, PPV, 1998, vol 1.

9 Andresen B: Persönlichkeitsstruktur und Psychosetendenz. Westerau, PPV, 1998, vol 2.
10 Becker P: Beyond the Big Five. Pers Individ Diff, in press.
11 McCrae RR: Psychopathology from the perspective of the Five-Factor Model; in Strack S, Lorr M (eds): Differentiating Normal and Abnormal Personality. New York, Springer, 1994, pp 26–39.
12 McCrae RR: A reformulation of axis II: Personality and personality-related problems; in Costa PT, Widiger TA (eds): Personality Disorders and the Five-Factor Model of Personality. Washington, American Psychological Association, 1994, pp 303–309.
13 Widiger TA, Sanderson CJ: Toward a dimensional model of personality disorders; in Livesley WJ (ed): The DSM-IV Personality Disorders. New York, Guilford Press, 1995, pp 433–458.
14 Wiggins JS, Pincus AL: Personality structure and the structure of personality disorders; in Costa PT, Widiger TA (eds): Personality Disorders and the Five-Factor Model of Personality. Washington, American Psychological Association 1994, pp 73–93.
15 Costa PT, McCrae RR: Personality disorders and the five-factor model of personality. J Pers Disord 1990;4:362–371.
16 Widiger TA, Trull TJ: Personality and psychopathology: An application of the Five-Factor Model. J Pers 1992;60:363–393.
17 Schroeder ML, Wormworth JA, Livesley WJ: Dimensions of personality disorder and their relationships to the Big Five dimensions of personality. Psychol Assess 1992;4:47–53.
18 Soldz S, Budman S, Demby A, Merry J: Representation of personality disorders in circumplex and five-factor space: Explorations with a clinical sample. Psychol Assess 1993;5:41–52.
19 Yeung AS, Lyons MJ, Waternaux CM, Faraone SV, Tsuang MT: The relationship between DSM-III personality disorders and the five-factor model of personality. Compr Psychiatry 1993;34:227–234.
20 Costa PT, Widiger TA (eds): Personality Disorders and the Five-Factor Model of Personality. Washington, American Psychological Association, 1994.
21 Dyce JA: Personality disorders: Alternatives to the official diagnostic system. J Pers Disord 1994;8:77–88.
22 American Psychiatric Association: Diagnostic and Statistical Manual of Mental Disorders, ed 4 rev. Washington, American Psychological Association, 1994.
23 Liddle PF: The symptoms of schizophrenia – A re-examination of the positive-negative dichotomy. Br J Psychiatry 1987;151:145–151.
24 Coolidge FL, Becker LA, DiRito DC, Durham RL, Kinlaw MM, Philbrick PB: On the relationship of the five-factor personality model to personality disorders: Four reservations. Psychol Rep 1994;75:11–21.
25 Clark LA, Vorhies L, McEven JL: Personality disorder symptomatology from the Five-Factor Model perspective; in Costa PT, Widiger TA (eds): Personality Disorders and the Five-Factor Model of Personality. Washington, American Psychological Association, 1994, pp 95–116.
26 Schroeder ML, Wormworth JA, Livesley WJ: Dimensions of personality disorder and the five factor model of personality; in Costa PT, Widiger TA (eds): Personality Disorders and the Five-Factor Model of Personality. Washington, American Psychological Association, 1994, pp 117–127.
27 Duijsens IJ, Diekstra RFW: DSM-III-R and ICD-10 personality disorders and their relationship with the Big Five dimensions of personality. Pers Individ Diff 1996;21:119–133.
28 Dyce JA, O'Connor BP: Personality disorders and the five-factor model: A test of facet-level predictions. J Pers Disord 1998;12:31–45.
29 Davis R, Millon T: On the importance of theory to a taxonomy of personality disorders; in Livesley WJ (ed): The DSM-IV Personality Disorders. New York, Guilford, 1995, pp 377–396.
30 Axelrod SR, Widiger TA, Trull TJ, Corbitt EM: Relations of Five-Factor Model antagonism facets with personality disorder symptomatology. J Pers Assess 1997;69:297–313.
31 Widiger TA: Categorial versus dimensional classification: Implications from and for research. J Pers Disord 1992;6:287–300.
32 Comrey AL, Schiebel D: Personality test correlates of psychiatric case history data. J Consult Clin Psychol 1985;53:470–479.
33 Craig RJ, Olson RE: Relationship between MCMI-II scales and normal personality traits. Psychol Rep 1992;71:699–705.
34 O'Boyle M, Holzer C: DSM-III-R personality disorders and Eysenck's personality dimensions. Pers Individ Diff 1992;13:1157–1159.
35 Svrakic DM, Whitehead C, Przybeck TR, Cloninger CR: Differential diagnosis of personality disorders by the Seven-Factor Model of temperament and character. Arch Gen Psychiatry 1993;50:991–999.
36 Goldman RG, Skodol AE, McGrath PJ, Oldham JM: Relationship between the tridimensional personality questionnaire and the DSM-III-R personality traits. Am J Psychiatry 1994; 151:274–276.
37 Mulder RT, Joyce PR: Temperament and the structure of personality disorder symptoms. Psychol Med 1997;27:99–106.
38 Westen D, Arkowitz-Westen L: Limitations of axis II in diagnosing personality pathology in clinical praxis. Am J Psychol 1998;155:1767–1771.
39 Zimmerman M, Coryell WH: DSM-III personality disorder dimensions. J Nerv Ment Dis 1990;178:686–692.
40 Schroeder ML, Livesley WJ: An evaluation of DSM-III-R personality disorders. Acta Psychiatr Scand 1991;84:512–519.
41 Bagby RM, Joffe RT, Parker JDA, Schuller DR: Re-examination of the evidence for the DSM-III personality disorder clusters. J Pers Disord 1993;7:320–328.
42 O'Connor BP, Dyce JA: A test of models of personality disorder configuration. J Abnorm Psychol 1998;107:3–16.
43 Livesley WJ, Jang KL, Vernon PA: Phenotypic and genetic structure of traits delineating personality disorder. Arch Gen Psychiatry 1998; 55:941–947.
44 Comrey AL: Comrey Personality Scales CPS, Manual. San Diego, Edits, 1987.
45 Cloninger CR, Svrakic DM, Przybeck TR: A psychobiological model of temperament and character. Arch Gen Psychiatry 1993;50:975–989.
46 Benet V, Waller NG: The Big Seven factor model of personality description: Evidence for its cross-cultural generality in a Spanish sample. J Pers Soc Psychol 1995;69:701–718.
47 Jackson DN, Paunonen SV, Fraboni M, Goffin RD: A five-factor versus six-factor model of personality structure. Pers Individ Diff 1996; 20:33–45.
48 Andresen B: Hamburger Persönlichkeits-Inventar HPI (Hamburg Personality Inventory HPI). Göttingen, Hogrefe, in press.
49 Costa PT, McCrae RR: The Five-Factor Model of personality and its relevance to personality disorders. J Pers Disord 1992;6:434–359.
50 Eysenck SBG, Eysenck HJ: The measurement of psychoticism: A study of factor stability and reliability. Br J Soc Clin Psychol 1968;7:286–294.
51 Eysenck SBG, Eysenck HJ, Barrett P: A revised version of the psychoticism scale. Pers Individ Diff 1985;6:21–29.
52 Goldberg LR, Rosolack TK: The Big Five Factor structure as an integrative framework: An empirical comparison with Eysenck's P-E-N model; in Halverson CF, Kohnstamm GA, Martin RP (eds): The Developing Structure of Temperament and Personality from Infancy to Adulthood. Hillsdale, Erlbaum, 1994, pp 7–35.
53 Klein C, Andresen B, Jahn T: Erfassung der schizotypen Persönlichkeit nach DSM-III-R (Assessment of schizotypal personality according to DSM-III-R). Diagnostica 1997;43:347–369.
54 Andresen B, Mass R (eds): Schizotypie – Psychometrische Entwicklungen und biopsychologische Forschungsansätze (Schizotypy – Psychometric Assessment and Psychobiological Research). Göttingen, Hogrefe, in press.
55 World Health Organisation: International Classification of Disease, Chapter V: Mental and Behavior Disorders, ed 10 rev. Geneva, World Health Organisation, 1992.
56 Borkenau P, Ostendorf F: Fünf-Faktoren-Inventar (NEO-FFI) nach Costa & McCrae (Five-Factor-Inventory (NEO-FFI) after Costa & McCrae), Manual. Göttingen, Hogrefe, 1993.
57 Hendriks AA, Hofstee WKB, DeRaad B, Goldberg LR, Angleitner A: The Five-Factor Personality Inventory (FFPI). Z Diff Diagn Psychol 1995;16:261.
58 Andresen B: Das Inventar Klinischer Persönlichkeitsakzentuierungen IKP (The Inventory of Clinical Personality Accentuations ICP). Göttingen, Hogrefe, in press.

59 Schneider K: Die psychopathischen Persönlichkeiten (The Psychopathic Personalities). Leipzig, Deuticke, 1934.
60 Fava JL, Velicer WF: An empirical comparison of factor, image, component, and scale scores. Multivariate Behav Res 1992;27:301–322.
61 Fava JL, Velicer WF: The effect of overextraction on factor and component analysis. Multivariate Behav Res 1992;27:387–415.
62 Pawlik K: Dimensionen des Verhaltens (Dimensions of Personality). Bern, Huber, 1968.
63 Trull TJ, Geary DC: Comparison of the big-five factor structure across samples of Chinese and American adults. J Pers Assess 1997;69: 324–341.
64 Costa PT, McCrae RR: Revised NEO Personality Inventory (NEO-PI-R) and NEO Five-Factor Inventory (NEO-FFI), Professional Manual. Odessa, Psychological Assessment Resources, 1992b.
65 Paulhus DL, Lysy DC, Yik MSM: Self-report measures of intelligence: Are they useful as proxy IQ tests? J Pers 1998;66:525–554.
66 Andresen B: Towards a comprehensive and unifying model of basic personality dimensions and personality disorder tendencies; in Mervielde I (ed): 8th European Conference on Personality, University of Ghent, Belgium, 8–12 July 1996, Abstracts. Gent, Academia Press, 1996, p 74.
67 Riemann R, Grubich C, Hempel S, Mergl S, Richter M: Personality and attitudes towards current political topics. Pers Individ Diff 1993; 15:313–321.
68 Wilson GD, Patterson JR: A new measure of conservatism. Br J Soc Clin Psychol 1968;7: 264–269.
69 Ostendorf F, Angleitner A: The structure of attitudes and its relation to the Big-Five factors of personality; in Mervielde I (ed): 8th European Conference on Personality, University of Ghent, Belgium, 8–12 July 1966, Abstracts. Gent, Academia Press, 1996, p 66.
70 Zerssen DV, Pfister H, Koeller D-M: The Munich Personality Test (MPT) – A short questionnaire for self-rating and relatives' rating of personality traits: Formal properties and clinical potential. Eur Arch Psychiatry Clin Neurosci 1988;238:73–93.
71 Andresen B, Stemmler G: Eine Dimensionsanalyse von 61 Persönlichkeitsskalen unter besonderer Berücksichtigung des Extraversions- und des Emotionalitätskomplexes (A dimensional analysis of 61 personality scales with special relevance of extraversion and neuroticism). Diagnostica 1982:28:340–347.
72 Andresen B: Differentielle Psychophysiologie valenzkonträrer Aktivierungsdimensionen (Differential Psychophysiology of Activation Dimensions with Opposite Emotional Valence). Frankfurt aM, Lang, 1987.
73 Glasberg HM, Bromberg PM, Stein M, Luparello TJ: A personality study of asthmatic patients. J Psychosom Res 1969;13:197–204.
74 Peabody D: Selecting representative trait adjectives. J Pers Soc Psychol 1987;52:59–71.
75 Lieshout CFMv, Haselager GJT: The Big Five personality factors in Q-sort descriptions of children and adolescents; in Halverson CF, Kohnstamm GA, Martin RP (eds): The Developing Structure of Temperament and Personality from Infancy to Adulthood. Hillsdale, Erlbaum, 1994, pp 293–318.
76 Jackson DN, Hourany L, Vidmar NJ: A four-dimensional interpretation of risk taking. J Pers 1972;40:483–501.
77 Bromiley P, Curley SP: Individual differences in risk taking; in Yates JF (ed): Risk Taking Behavior. Chichester, Wiley, 1992.
78 Krüger C, Amelang M: Bereitschaft zu riskantem Verhalten als Trait-Konstrukt und Test-Konzept: Zur Entwicklung eines Fragebogens auf der Basis des Handlungs-Häufigkeits-Ansatzes (Readiness to take risks as a trait construct and test concept: Development of a questionnaire on the basis of an act-frequency approach). Diagnostica 1995;41:35–52.
79 Zuckerman M: Sensation seeking and risk taking; in Izard CE (ed): Emotions in Personality and Psychopathology. New York, Plenum, 1980, pp 163–197.
80 Andresen B: Reizsuche- und Erlebnismotive II: Sekundärfaktoranalysen, Invarianzprüfung und Ableitung eines MISAP-Strukturmodells (Sensation and experience-seeking motives II: Second order factor analyses, judgement of invariance and proposal of a structural model for MISAP). Z Diff Diagn Psychol 1990;11:65–92.
81 Zuckerman M, Eysenck SBG, Eysenck HJ: Sensation seeking in England and America: Cross-cultural, age, and sex comparisons. J Consult Clin Psychol 1978;46:139–149.
82 Zuckerman M, Kuhlman DM, Thornquist M, Kiers H: Five (or three) robust questionnaire scale factors of personality without culture. Pers Individ Diff 1991;12:929–941.
83 Zuckerman M, Kuhlman DM, Joireman J, Teta P, Kraft M: A comparison of the three structural models for personality: The Big Three, the Big Five, and the Alternative Five. J Pers Soc Psychol 1993;65:757–768.
84 Zuckerman M: Psychobiology of Personality. New York, Cambridge University Press, 1991.
85 Tellegen A: Folk concepts and psychological concepts of personality and personality disorder. Psychol Inquiry 1993;4:122–130.
86 Saucier G, Goldberg LR: What is beyond the Big Five? J Pers 1998;66:495–524.
87 Widiger TA: Conceptualizing a disorder of personality from the Five-Factor Model; in Costa PT, Widiger TA (eds): Personality Disorders and the Five-Factor Model of Personality. Washington, American Psychological Association, 1994, pp 311–317.
88 Nakao K, Gunderson JG, Phillips KA, Tanaka N, Yorifuji K, Takaishi J, Nishimura T: Functional impairment in personality disorders. J Pers Disord 1992;6:24–33.
89 Zimmerman M, Coryell W: DSM-III personality disorder diagnoses in a nonpatient sample. Arch Gen Psychiatry 1989;46:682–689.
90 Tyrer P, Gunderson J, Lyons M, Tohen M: Special feature: Extent of comorbidity between mental state and personality disorders. J Pers Disord 1997;11:242–259.
91 Skodol AE, Rosnick L, Kellman D, Oldham JM, Hyler SE: Validating structured DSM-III-R personality disorder assessment with longitudinal data. Am J Psychiatry 1988;145: 1297–1299.
92 Millon T: Personality disorders: Conceptual distinctions and classification issues; in Costa PT, Widiger TA (eds): Personality Disorders and the Five-Factor Model of Personality. Washington, American Psychological Association, 1994, pp 279–301.
93 Tellegen A, Lykken DT, Bouchard TJ, Wilcox KJ, Segal NL, Rich S: Personality similarity in twins reared apart and together. J Pers Soc Psychol 1988;54:1031–1039.
94 Francis LJ, Brown LB, Lester D, Philipchalk R: Happiness as stable extraversion: A cross-cultural examination of the reliability and validity of the Oxford Happiness Inventory among students in the UK, USA, Australia, and Canada. Pers Individ Diff 1998;24:167–171.
95 Jenkins TN: Measurement of the primary factors of total personality. J Psychol 1962;54: 417–442.
96 Stemmler G: Differential Psychophysiology: Persons in Situations. New York, Springer, 1992.
97 Eysenck HJ: The Biological Basis of Personality. Springfield, Thomas, 1967.
98 Brocke B, Tasche KG, Beauducel A: Biopsychological foundations of extraversion: Differential effort reactivity and state control. Pers Individ Diff 1997;22:447–458.
99 Brocke B, Tasche KG, Beauducel A: Biopsychological foundations of extraversion: Differential effort reactivity and the differential P300 effect. Pers Individ Diff 1996;21:727–738.
100 Debus G, Erdmann G, Kallus KW (eds): Biopsychologie von Stress und emotionalen Reaktionen (Biopsychology of stress and emotional reactions). Göttingen, Hogrefe, 1995.
101 Janke W, Debus G: Double-blind psychometric evaluation of pimozide and haloperidol versus placebo in emotionally labile volunteers under two different work load conditions. Pharm-Psychiatr – Neur-Psychopharmakol 1972;5:34–51.
102 Smokler IA, Shevrin H: Cerebral lateralization and personality style. Arch Gen Psychiatry 1979;36:949–954.
103 Tomarken AJ, Davidson RJ: Frontal brain activation in repressors and nonrepressors. J Abnorm Psychol 1994;103:339–349.
104 Ernst AM: Digest: Kooperation und Konkurrenz (Digest: Cooperation and competition): Spektrum der Wissenschaft. Digest 1998;1:6.
105 Curtin F, Walker J-P, Peyrin L, Soulier V, Badan M, Schulz P: Reward dependence is positively related to urinary monoamines in normal men. Biol Psychiatry 1997;42:275–281.

106 Netter-Munkelt P: Psychometrische Studien zur psychophysischen Geschlechtskonstitution (Psychometric studies on psychophysical constitution of gender). Psychol Beitr 1972; 14:124–156.
107 Dabbs JM, Hargrove MF, Heusel C: Testosterone differences among college fraternities: Well behaved vs rambunctious. Pers Individ Diff 1996;20:157–161.
108 Schwartz GE, Brown S-L, Ahern GL: Facial muscle patterning and subjective experience during affective imagery: Sex differences. Psychophysiology 1980;17:75–82.
109 Clark LA, Livesley WJ: Two approaches to identifying the dimensions of personality disorders: Convergence on the Five-Factor Model; in Costa PT, Widiger TA (eds): Personality Disorders and the Five-Factor Model of Personality. Washington, American Psychological Association, 1994, pp 261–277.
110 Pukrop R, Herpertz S, Sass H, Steinmeyer EM: Special feature: Personality and personality disorders. A facet theoretical analysis of the similarity relationships. J Pers Disord 1998;12:226–246.
111 Gelernter J, Kranzler H, Coccaro EF, Siever LJ, New AS: Serotonin transporter protein gene polymorphism and personality measures in African American and European American subjects. Am J Psychiatry 1998;155:1332–1338.
112 Wang S, Mason J, Charney D, Yehuda R, Riney S, Southwick S: Relationships between hormonal profile and novelty seeking in combat-related posttraumatic stress disorder. Biol Psychiatry 1997;41:145–151.
113 Askenazy F, Candito M, Caci H, Myquel M, Chambon P, Darcourt G, Puech AJ: Whole blood serotonin content, tryptophan concentrations, and impulsivity in anorexia nervosa. Biol Psychiatry 1998;43:188–195.
114 O'Connor TG, McGuire S, Reiss D, Hetherington EM, Plomin R: Co-occurrence of depressive symptoms and antisocial behavior in adolescence: A common genetic liability. J Abnorm Psychol 1998;107:27–37.
115 Wills TA, Windle M, Cleary SD: Temperament and novelty seeking in adolescent substance use: Convergence of dimensions of temperament with constructs from Cloninger's theory. J Pers Soc Psychol 1998;74:387–406.
116 Fahrenberg J: Concepts of activation and arousal in the theory of emotionality (neuroticism); in Strelau J, Eysenck HJ (eds): Personality Dimensions and Arousal. New York, Plenum Press, 1987.
117 Heath AC, Cloninger CR, Martin NG: Testing a model for the genetic structure of personality: A comparison of the personality systems of Cloninger and Eysenck. J Pers Soc Psychol 1994;66:762–775.
118 Bergeman CS, Chipuer HM, Plomin R, Pedersen NL, McClearn GE, Nesselroade JR, Costa PT, McCrae RR: Genetic and environmental effects on openness to experience, agreeableness, and conscientiousness: An adoption/twin study. J Pers 1993;61:159–179.
119 McGuffin P, Thapar A: The genetics of personality disorder. Br J Psychiatry 1992;160: 12–23.
120 Dahl AA: The personality disorders: A critical review of family, twin, and adoption studies. J Pers Disord 1993;suppl spring:86–99.
121 Livesley WJ, Jang KL, Jackson DN, Vernon PA: Genetic and environmental contributions to dimensions of personality disorder. Am J Psychiatry 1993;150:1826–1831.
122 Paris J: Personality disorders: A biopsychosocial model. J Pers Disord 1993;7:255–264.
123 Torgerson S, Skre I, Onstad S, Edvardsen J, Kringlen E: The psychometric-genetic structure of DSM-III-R personality disorder criteria. J Pers Disord 1993;7:196–213.
124 Parker G: Special feature: The etiology of personality disorders: A review and consideration of research models. J Pers Disord 1997; 11:345–369.

Neuropsychobiology

Neuropsychobiology 2000;41:24–30

Sensation Seeking and Affective Disorders: Characteristics in the Intensity Dependence of Acoustic Evoked Potentials

Burkhard Brocke[a] André Beauducel[a] Regina John[a] Stefan Debener[a]
Hubert Heilemann[b]

[a]Institute of Psychology II, Dresden University of Technology, Dresden, and
[b]State Mental Hospital Arnsdorf, Germany

Key Words

Bipolar affective disorder · Unipolar affective disorder · Sensation seeking · Augmenting/reducing

Abstract

Augmenting/reducing of the evoked potential has been shown to be related to sensation seeking (SS) and specific clinical disorders. Buchsbaum demonstrated that patients with bipolar affective disorders (BAD) tend to be augmenters, as is the case with sensation seekers, and patients with unipolar affective disorders (UPD) tend to be reducers. In addition, he reported that prophylactic medication reduced the tendency to augment in bipolar patients. However, evidence for these relations is restricted to a few studies. This study explores whether Buchsbaum's initial findings can be found in a naturalistic clinical setting. Acoustic evoked potentials were recorded for six levels of intensity (59, 71, 79, 88, 92, 96 dB SPL) from 24 healthy adults, 21 unipolar depressed patients, and 21 patients with BAD. Participants also completed personality questionnaires, especially the Sensation Seeking Scales Form V. Results revealed a positive correlation between SS and augmenting/reducing in healthy controls, thereby replicating earlier findings. Bipolar depressed patients showed larger P1/N1 slopes than healthy controls, when medication was statistically controlled. Unipolar depressed patients showed smaller P2 slopes, but only when medication was not controlled. Implications of these results for further research on augmenting/reducing and affective disorders and their relationship to SS are discussed.

Introduction

A number of findings suggest a positive relation between sensation seeking (SS) and the augmenting disposition of the evoked potential (EP) of the EEG [1]. When stimulus intensity increases, sensation seekers respond with a marked increase in the P1/N1 or N1/P2 component of the EP. This change is also referred to as augmenting disposition or 'high-level intensity dependence'. Since Zuckerman's [1] review, this finding has been replicated several times [2, 3]. In a recent study, we could also confirm the correlation between SS and augmenting [4]. However, some of the inconsistencies in the earlier findings still require clarification. Methodological problems concern the lack of comparability of various EP parameters that were used [5].

There are indications that particularities of the intensity dependence also appear in certain psychological disorders, for instance in alcoholism and affective disorders [6, 7]. Following the basic work by Buchsbaum et al. [6], several studies found that patients with bipolar affective dis-

KARGER

Fax + 41 61 306 12 34
E-Mail karger@karger.ch
www.karger.com

0302–282X/00/0411–0024$17.50/0

Accessible online at:
www.karger.com/journals/nps

Prof. Dr. Burkhard Brocke
TU Dresden, Institut für Psychologie II
Mommsenstrasse 13
D–01062 Dresden (Germany)
E-Mail brocke@rcs.urz.tu-dresden.de

orders (BAD) show a pronounced augmenting disposition in comparison to healthy controls. Another finding is that responders to antidepressant or prophylactic medication are augmenters, whereas nonresponders tend to be reducers [7, 8]. With regard to unipolar depression (UPD), Buchsbaum's findings suggest that these patients exhibit a significantly lower intensity dependence than did BAD patients and healthy controls, thereby showing themselves to be reducers [9].

Thus far, several findings suggest that sensation seekers (SS) and BAD share psychophysiological characteristics, and SS and UPD patients might differ with regard to augmenting/reducing. This relationship could turn out to be mutually indicative of the SS trait and affective disorders if further findings support the assumption that a high level of intensity dependence in EP can be taken as an indicator of low central serotonergic neurotransmission, particularly in the primary auditory cortex [7]. Peculiarities of central serotonergic neurotransmission are assumed to be of importance for both SS and affective disorders [7, 10].

In addition, the question arises as to whether BAD and SS are also associated behaviorally or psychometrically, and in particular whether SS might be a vulnerability factor for the development of a bipolar disorder. The psychophysiological findings described thus far support this assumption and correspond well with initial psychometric findings on the relation between SS and affective disorders. Using the SS Scale Form V (SSS-V) [11], Zuckerman and Neeb [12] were able to distinguish between controls and patients with a reported history of bipolar depression. Cronin and Zuckerman [13] showed that inpatients with bipolar depression had significantly higher SS scores (subscales disinhibition and boredom susceptibility) than controls, though half of the patients were depressed at the time of the study.

Little is known about the effects of antidepressant and prophylactic medication with serotonergic relevance on the augmenting/reducing characteristic of BAD and UPD. The study by Buchsbaum et al. [6] revealed a significant decrease in the intensity dependence of BAD under lithium ('flattening effect'). Some studies found the same effect on the intensity dependence for different patient groups when tricyclic antidepressants and selective serotonin reuptake inhibitors (SSRI) were used [14, 15, summarized in 7]. Overall, it has not been clarified yet whether the flattening effect is stable or only transient during the first time of medication, since appropriate studies with retests over a respective period are not available. Thus, the question arises whether the stronger intensity dependence of BAD patients compared to healthy controls under antidepressant or prophylactic medication really changes in favor of a flattening effect, and whether the intensity dependence of both groups is similar under these conditions.

The study by Buchsbaum et al. [6] does not give evidence of changes on the intensity dependence of unipolar depressed patients while treated with lithium. So far, studies on the effect of antidepressant medication with UPD patients have been mainly restricted to clinical responsiveness studies [8, 16].

All in all, the actual findings concerning the intensity dependence of antidepressant or prophylactically medicated BAD and UPD patients in comparison to healthy controls do not offer sufficient information yet. The present study investigates the intensity dependence of SS in healthy individuals. In addition, the aim of the study was to investigate differences in the intensity dependence between both affective-disordered groups (BAD, UPD) and in comparison to healthy individuals. At the psychometric level, it is attempted to replicate the findings of higher SS scores for BAD and lower SS scores for UPD when compared to controls.

Methods

Participants

Inpatients with diagnoses of affective disorders were recruited from the State Mental Hospital Arnsdorf, Germany. Patients' participation did not interfere with their therapeutic treatment. Hospital staff and interested volunteers were recruited as controls (n = 24; age: mean = 47, SD = 11; 16 females) and screened for current or past history of psychiatric illness and substance abuse. Written informed consent was obtained from all participants.

A structured clinical interview [17] was taken by a trained graduate student, and consensus diagnosis was established together with an experienced psychiatrist (H.H.). Patients with ambiguous diagnoses (n = 17) were not included in the analysis. Furthermore, patients were excluded if they had a past history of organic brain disorder or substance abuse (n = 5). We obtained EEG retest data from 27 of the final sample of 42 patients.

According to the International Classification of Diseases [18], 21 patients of the final sample were diagnosed as suffering from UPD (age: mean = 47, SD = 11; 12 females); of these, 20 patients were classified as having a depressive episode (F32), and 1 patient as having a recurrent depressive disorder (F33). The second clinical group consisted of 21 patients with a diagnosis of BAD, who were in different episodes at the recording time (BAD; F31; age: mean = 43, SD = 12; 8 females). Seven of the 21 BAD patients had psychotic symptoms, whereas none of the UPD patients had psychotic symptoms during the time period of the study. There were no significant differences in age and gender distributions between BAD, UPD and the control group.

Medication status for all patients was monitored over the interval of the study. The majority of the UPD patients received antidepressant medication (13 tricyclic antidepressants, 3 SSRI). Two patients received prophylactic medication (lithium), 2 neuroleptic medication. One patient received anxiolytic medication only, whereas 12 patients received anxiolytic comedication (benzodiazepines). One UPD patient was unmedicated.

The BAD patients received prophylactic (9 lithium, 5 carbamazepine) or antidepressant medication (3 tricyclic antidepressants, 3 SSRI). Two of them received both antidepressant and prophylactic medication and 12 anxiolytic or neuroleptic medication as comedication.

Participants were requested to fill in self-report personality questionnaires. Special interest was focused on the SSS-V [11] which consists of the four subscales thrill and adventure seeking (TAS), disinhibiton (DIS), experience seeking (ES), and boredom susceptibility (BS).

Data Collection and Quantification

In order to check the stability of the EEG measurements, a retest was scheduled 2–4 weeks after the initial recording session. Separate diagnostic sessions, including the assessment of personality dimensions and clinical state, were scheduled within a few days of the EEG recording sessions. All recordings were scheduled at fixed times and intervals in the morning.

After audiometric screening of participants, EEG data were recorded from 19 standard scalp sites (10–20 system) using a forehead ground and linked earlobes as reference, while participants sat in a comfortable arm chair with their eyes open. EEG data were band pass filtered (0.1–30 Hz) and continuously digitized at 256 samples/s. To facilitate artifact rejection, the vertical electro-oculogram was recorded from additional electrodes placed above and below the right eye. After a recording of 8 min of resting EEG, the acoustic augmenting/reducing paradigm [19] was administered (13 min time duration). For a more accurate calculation of the intensity dependence, six different intensity levels were used (59, 71, 79, 88, 92, 96 dB SPL). Stimuli were presented binaurally via headphones in a pseudorandomized order. Each 1,000-Hz stimulus lasted 30 ms (10 ms each of rise and fall time), the interstimulus interval varied between 1,600 and 2,100 ms.

EEG data were epoched off-line from 100 ms before to 400 ms after stimulus onset. Following baseline correction of the prestimulus interval to 0 μV, epochs with artifacts were excluded automatically if the EEG signal exceeded ±50 μV prestimulus or ±65 μV poststimulus. Long-latency acoustic EP (AEP) were obtained by averaging the remaining epochs for each stimulus intensity separately (minimum sweep number 20 epochs). Peak amplitudes were determined for the P1 as the most positive peak within the period of 25–80 ms, for the N1 as the most negative peak within 55–135 ms, and for P2 as the most positive peak within 110–260 ms. Additional peak-to-peak values were calculated for P1/N1 and N1/P2.

Statistical Analysis

Similar to previous studies, the slopes of the linear regression line (least-squares technique) for the individual P1, N1, P2, P1/N1 and N1/P2 amplitudes were calculated across the six stimulus intensities. However, because the use of regression slopes for the amplitude stimulus intensity function (ASF) has been criticized for their low coefficients of determination in individual data [20], a nonlinear computation was also performed [2]. The medians of all possible slopes between each two amplitudes for the six stimulus intensities (median slopes) were calculated. All parameters were calculated for C3, Cz and C4 scalp locations [1].

Table 1. Retest reliabilities of the augmenting/reducing parameters in controls and patients for ASF slopes and median slopes at three central scalp sites, separately

Parameters	ASF slopes			Median slopes		
	C3	Cz	C4	C3	Cz	C4
Controls (n = 24)						
P1	0.18	0.02	0.14	0.04	–0.08	–0.08
N1	0.38	0.07	0.06	0.08	–0.27	–0.01
P2	*0.61*	*0.77*	*0.67*	*0.47*	*0.65*	*0.50*
P1/N1	0.19	0.30	0.31	0.27	0.17	*0.50*
N1/P2	*0.77*	*0.71*	*0.59*	*0.79*	*0.80*	*0.64*
Patients (n = 28)						
P1	0.20	0.25	*0.43*	0.24	0.34	0.29
N1	*0.53*	*0.58*	0.21	*0.53*	*0.41*	0.28
P2	*0.41*	*0.61*	*0.47*	0.23	*0.42*	0.17
P1/N1	0.22	0.34	0.17	*0.41*	*0.43*	*0.43*
N1/P2	0.17	0.38	0.18	0.03	0.22	0.11

Pearson correlations >0.40 are in italics.

Preliminary analyses addressed the retest reliability of the different computations of augmenting/reducing to evaluate effects of electrode site, AEP components, and the method of parametrization for patients and healthy controls separately. A second recording session was available from 14 BAD, 14 UPD and 24 control participants. Additional correlational analyses focused on the relationship of the augmenting/reducing tendency with the SS trait for healthy participants only.

To examine the group differences in augmenting/reducing, data from the first recording session were submitted to a 2 × 3 repeated-measures analysis of variance (ANOVA), including position (C3, Cz, C4) and group. Since we assumed different effects comparing UPD, BAD and controls, the group differences were tested separately. Additional analyses included session as a repeated-measures factor for those participants where a retest was available. Comparisons for all pairs of groups (UPD vs. controls, BAD vs. controls, UPD vs. BAD) are reported for ASF slopes only, because analyses for median slopes revealed similar results.

To be sure that no group effects are interpreted that may be related to the effects of antidepressants, medication effects were controlled by means of covariates. The applied medications were coded as yes (1) or no (0). However, the influence of the covariates is not independent of the frequency of the medication applied. The total number of participants receiving partially similar medication is different for the UPD and BAD groups. Therefore, it is important to control for medication, in order to control for effects due to different frequencies of medication in the groups. The covariates represent the direct influence of a medication on augmenting/reducing together with the frequency of the respective medication and therefore have to be interpreted with caution.

Differences in SS between UPD, BAD and controls were calculated by means of t tests, for the SSS-V total scale and the four subscales.

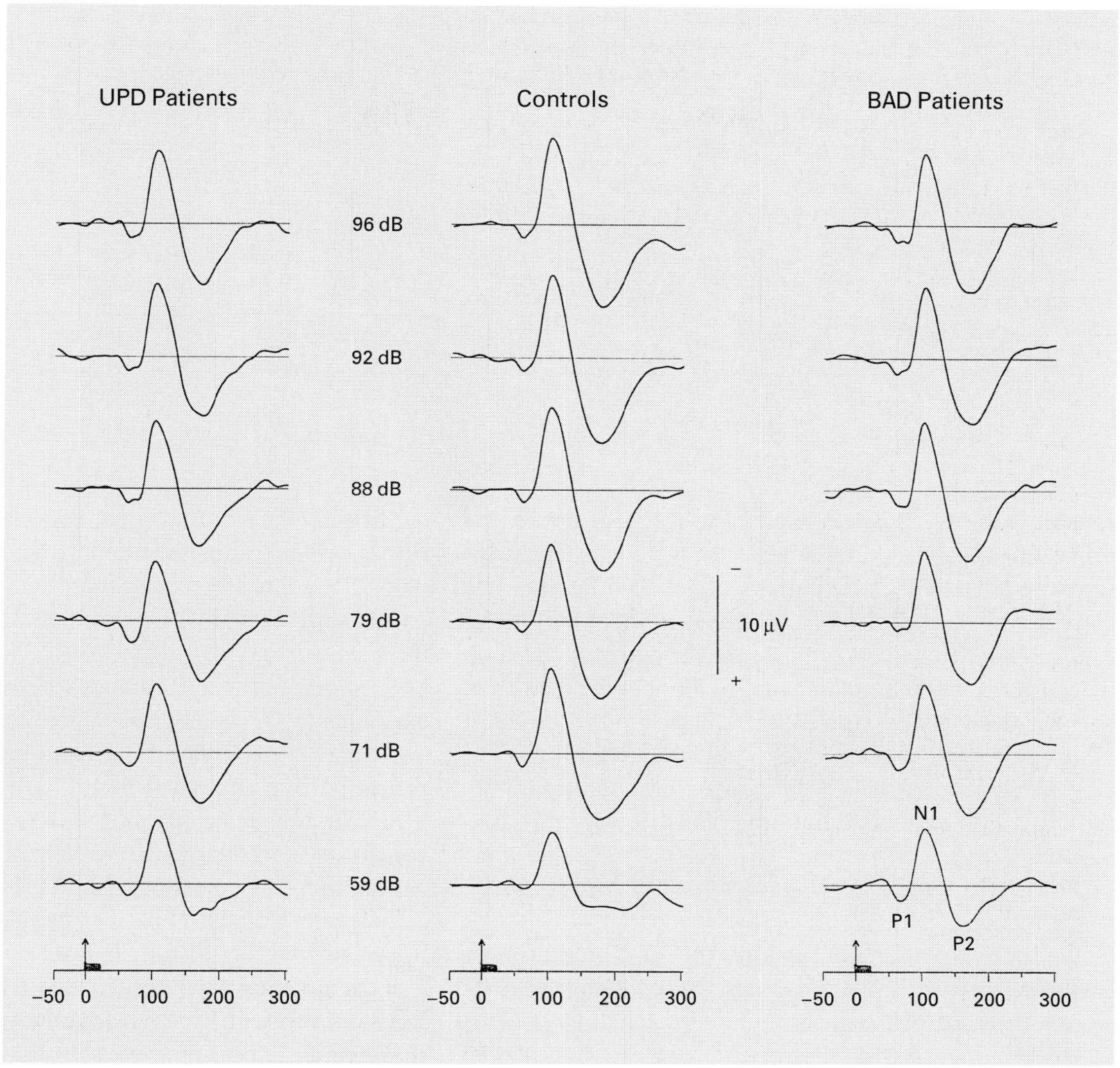

Fig. 1. Grand average AEP for UPD patients (n = 21), patients with BAD (n = 21), and healthy controls (n = 24) for six different stimulus intensities at recording site Cz. The AEP components P1, N1 and P2 are indicated for BAD patients at 59 dB SPL.

Results

Figure 1 shows the AEP for the scalp site Cz for UPD patients (left column), healthy controls (middle column) and BAD patients (right column). Averages are separately displayed for each stimulus intensity level from 59 dB (bottom) up to 96 dB (top). Independent of group, the P1, N1, and P2 components of the AEP were apparent at each level of stimulus intensity. Overall, the augmenting tendency was visible in each group, i.e. a pronounced amplitude increase with increasing stimulus intensity.

Reliability of the AEP Parameters (Intensity Dependence)

The following test-retest reliabilities (temporal stability) were computed for the control group (n = 24) and the patient group (n = 28) separately. The retest reliabilities for the parameters differed considerably in both patients and controls (table 1).

For controls, satisfactory retest reliabilities were achieved for the ASF slopes for P2 and N1/P2, irrespective of the electrode site. The slopes of the linear regression line for the P1, N1, and P1/N1 amplitudes were not

Table 2. Pearson correlations of the ASF slopes with the SSS-V total score in controls (n = 24)

Parameters	First recording session			Second recording session			Aggregated across sessions		
	C3	Cz	C4	C3	Cz	C4	C3	Cz	C4
P1	0.34	0.27	0.29	0.11	0.15	0.26	0.29	0.30	0.37*
N1	0.30	0.30	0.37*	0.12	0.04	0.22	0.24	0.20	0.40*
P2	0.29	0.37*	0.35*	0.45*	0.34*	0.41*	0.41*	0.38*	0.42*
P1/N1	0.01	–0.01	–0.10	–0.04	0.08	–0.01	–0.02	0.04	–0.06
N1/P2	0.07	0.16	0.00	0.27	0.23	0.16	0.18	0.21	0.09

* $p < 0.05$, one tailed.

reliable (table 1). When compared to the ASF slopes, the reliabilities of the median slopes were not consistently different. For patients, the pattern of reliabilities was less consistent in comparison to healthy participants. Whereas the N1/P2 slope was not reliable for patients, acceptable values were obtained for the N1 slopes on C3 and Cz, and for the P2 slopes on all sites. The pattern of retest reliabilities was different for ASF slopes and median slopes. However, across both groups, method of parametrization did not affect reliabilities consistently.

SS and Intensity Dependence of the AEP for Healthy Participants

On both measurement sessions, the most obvious relationships with the SSS-V total score were found for the P2 slopes, the parameters with the highest reliabilities. This result remained stable when measurements were pooled across sessions. The SSS-V total score correlated with the P2 slopes, which were reliable, but it correlated only inconsistently with the P1 and N1 slopes (table 2). P1 and N1 slopes were not reliable in healthy participants. For the N1/P2, only a correlation with the SSS-V subscale TAS was found ($r = 0.36$, $p < 0.05$, one tailed) on C3 in the second recording session. Pooled across sessions, the slopes of the P1 and N1 on C4 showed significant relations with the SSS-V total score. Since the correlations of P1 and N1 slopes with SSS-V scores indicated some validity of these parameters, we included them into further analyses. The expected positive correlation between SS and the intensity dependence of the AEP was confirmed again by the present results.

Clinical Groups and Intensity Dependence

For the first session, a significant main effect was found for P1/N1 slopes, when controlled for medication, confirming the assumption of BAD patients having larger slopes, when compared to controls, $F(1, 37) = 5.91$, $p < 0.05$. The same effect remained significant without BAD patients medicated with neuroleptics, when controlled for medication, $F(1, 30) = 8.50$, $p < 0.01$. Similarly, a tendency was found for the P1 slopes when controlled for medication, $F(1, 37) = 3.88$, $p = 0.056$.

For UPD patients compared to healthy controls, a significant group effect was found between the P2 slopes of UPD patients and controls, $F(1, 43) = 5.91$, $p < 0.05$, with controls having a larger slope. When controlled for medication, this effect disappeared, $F(1, 38) = 1.34$, n.s. Calculated without the UPD patients treated with neuroleptics, the effect was significant, $F(1, 41) = 5.69$, $p < 0.05$, but also disappeared when controlled for medication, $F(1, 37) = 0.74$, n.s. A tendency was found for groups when N1/P2 slopes of UPD patients were compared to controls. Again, UPD patients had smaller slopes when compared to healthy controls, $F(1, 43) = 3.68$, $p = 0.062$. This tendency was not significant when controlled for medication, $F(1, 38) = 0.42$, n.s. Without the UPD patients treated with neuroleptics, there was a similar tendency for the N1/P2 slopes, $F(1, 41) = 3.18$, $p = 0.082$, which disappeared when controlled for medication, $F(1, 37) = 0.00$, n.s. The effects of the covariates for tricyclic antidepressive drugs and SSRI were mainly responsible for this shift.

For the first recording session, none of the comparisons between BAD patients and UPD patients reached significance, even when controlled for medication.

In the ANOVAs for patients with two AEP recording sessions (15 with UPD, 12 with BAD), there was only a main effect for UPD patients having smaller N1/P2 slopes than controls, $F(1, 37) = 5.01$, $p < 0.05$. A similar main effect for the P2 slopes occurred, $F(1, 37) = 4.90$, $p <$

0.05. No main effect for recording session nor any group × session interaction was found. Despite of changes in the therapeutic medication of several patients, the effects remained stable across the recording sessions.

Clinical Groups and SS

As expected, BAD patients had significantly higher SSS-V total scores than UPD patients, $t = -2.29$, $p < 0.05$ (this and the following significances reflect one-tailed tests). BAD patients scored significantly higher than UPD patients on the subscales ES, $t = -2.30$, $p < 0.05$, and DIS, $t = -2.89$, $p < 0.01$. In addition, BAD patients had greater SSS-V total scores than controls, $t = -1.80$, $p < 0.05$, and scored higher on the DIS subscale, $t = -2.59$, $p < 0.05$. For the differences between UPD patients and controls, there was – again in accordance with the assumptions – a tendency for ES, $t = 1.43$, $p = 0.08$, with UPD patients scoring lower.

The confirmed relationship of SS with ASF slopes in healthy participants, as well as significant group differences in SS, may have modulated group differences for ASF slopes. We therefore reanalyzed our data. The corresponding position × group × SS ANOVA was based on a median split of the SSS-V total score of group-specific medians. These analyses did not reveal any significant interaction involving SS for either the first or the second recording session.

Discussion

At the psychophysiological level, we were again able to replicate the positive correlation between augmenting and SS [4, 10]. These findings are especially informative since the study yields data on the reliabilities of the parameters used. The correlations with SS were again confirmed for the P2 slopes in healthy participants. This result may be due to remarkable reliabilities of this parameter. However, the N1/P2 slopes, which showed comparable reliabilities, only correlated with the TAS subscale. For healthy participants, inconsistent correlations of the N1 and P2 slopes with SS emerged. This goes parallel with low reliabilities of the N1 and P2 slopes in this study.

In addition, we found the expected steeper ASF slopes for BAD patients, i.e. augmenting, when controlled for medication. Without controlling for medication, no effects reached significance for ASF slopes. Thus, it is possible that the medication of the BAD patients flattens the slopes, and therefore eleminates the differences between BAD patients and controls [6, 7]. When calculated without patients with neuroleptic medication, the results remained similar, so that the flattening effect may not be due to neuroleptic medication. However, further studies with more homogeneously medicated patients are necessary in order to assess the influence of different types of medication on individual differences in ASF slopes.

Our results indicate that UPD patients have smaller ASF slopes than controls, but this does not hold when controlled for medication. This means that the medication of the UPD patients could be responsible for their smaller ASF slopes. On the other hand, it might be possible that UPD patients would still have smaller slopes without medication, as reported by Buchsbaum et al. [6]. The analyses across recording sessions point into this direction because UPD patients have smaller ASF slopes than controls even when medication changes. The changes in medication in UPD patients across recording sessions had no effect on the ASF slopes since there was no significant change in the slopes across sessions. This, furthermore, indicates that the smaller slope of the UPD patients cannot be totally attributed to the effects of medication.

Overall, the results must be regarded with caution, because it was only possible to control medication effects on the augmenting/reducing disposition by means of statistical analysis. Even if equal group size for every type of medication and comedication could be obtained, there will always be confounding influences left (e.g. type of disease and medication), which cannot be completely controlled for. However, these limitations are typically given in naturalistic settings, since it is neither possible nor recommended to leave patients unmedicated.

At the psychometric level, the differences in SSS-V scores confirmed our assumption of BAD patients having higher scores than UPD patients and controls. This is a further replication of the results of Zuckerman and Neeb [12], Cronin and Zuckerman [13] and Carton et al. [21]. Some of the results of Carton et al. [21] could only be replicated with reservations, because there was only a tendency for the difference between UPD patients and controls. However, SS did not modulate group differences in ASF slopes, as revealed by reanalyses. The group-specific differences in SS did not account for additional variance in ASF slopes. This finding suggests that group characteristics and SS are highly dependent and that they account for a large amount of common variance in ASF slopes.

Overall, some psychophysiological and psychometric differences between BAD and UPD patients and controls could be demonstrated, which were in line with the few findings on these relations when controlled for medication. In addition, when effects of prophylactic or antidepressant medication are not statistically controlled, the relations are also compatible with the reported characteristics of the intensity dependence of medicated BAD, i.e. the flattening effect of the slopes when medicated. However, due to the naturalistic setting of this study, these results must be taken with caution and can only be seen as an indication. Future studies, especially with more restricted medication or with pre/postdesigns, are needed for further clarification of the characteristic intensity dependence of unmedicated BAD and UPD patients and the effects of antidepressant and prophylactic medication on these groups. However, this is not easily accomplished. Besides, the prognostic value of SS and augmenting/reducing in the clinical context might be more appropriately assessed in a naturalistic setting.

Acknowledgments

We are grateful to A. Naumann, D. Nessler, S. Raabe and D. Schulze for their help in testing. We also acknowledge the technical support by J. Schäfer, G. Pascher and V. Hantzsch, and thank C.L. Brown for additional software support.

References

1 Zuckerman M: The psychophysiology of sensation seeking. J Pers 1990;58:313–345.
2 Hegerl U, Karnauchow I, Herrmann WM, Müller-Oerlinghausen B: Intensity dependence of auditory evoked N1/P2 component and personality. Neuropsychobiology 1992:26:166–172.
3 Hegerl U, Gallinat J, Mrowinski D: Sensory cortical processing and the biological basis of personality. Biol Psychiatry 1995;37:467–472.
4 Brocke B, Beauducel A, Tasche K: Biopsychological bases and behavioral correlates of sensation seeking: Contributions to a multilevel validation. Pers Individ Diff 1999;26:1103–1123.
5 Beauducel A, Debener S, Brocke B: Methodological issues of the augmenting/reducing paradigm: Retest-reliability of different parameters suggest the need to identify mediating factors (abstract). J Psychophysiol, in press.
6 Buchsbaum MS, Goodwin F, Murphy D, Borge G: AER in affective disorders. Am J Psychiatry 1971;128:19–25.
7 Hegerl U, Juckel G: Intensity dependence of auditory evoked potentials as an indicator of central serotonergic neurotransmission: A new hypothesis. Biol Psychiatry 1993;33:173–187.
8 Hegerl U, Herrmann, WM: Event-related potentials and the prediction of differential drug response in psychiatry. Neuropsychobiology 1990;23:99–108.
9 Kang J, Fitzpatrick DF, Kline JP, Hendricks SE, Graber B: Average evoked potential response augmentation/reduction: Correlates and alteration with antidepressant therapy. Biol Psychiatry 1991;29:2058.
10 Zuckerman M: Behavioral Expressions and Biological Bases of Sensation Seeking. New York, Cambridge University Press, 1994.
11 Zuckerman M, Eysenck S, Eysenck HJ: Sensation seeking in England and America: Cross-cultural, age and sex comparisons. J Consult Clin Psychol 1978;46:139–149.
12 Zuckerman M, Neeb M: Sensation seeking and psychopathology. Psychiatry Res 1979;1:255–264.
13 Cronin C, Zuckerman M: Sensation seeking and bipolar affective disorder. Pers Individ Diff 1992;13:385–387.
14 Von Knorring L, Johansson F, Almay B: Augmenting/reducing response in visual evoked potentials in patients with chronic pain syndromes. Adv Biol Psychiatry 1980;4:55–62.
15 Von Knorring L: Effect of imipramine and zimelidine on the augmenting-reducing response of visual-evoked potentials in healthy volunteers. Adv Biol Psychiatry 1982;9:81–86.
16 Paige SR, Fitzpatrick DF, Kline JP, Balogh SE, Hendricks SE: Event-related potential amplitude intensity slopes predict response to antidepressants. Neuropsychobiology 1994;30: 197–201.
17 Pfister H, Wittchen H, Weigel A: Composite International Diagnostic Interview (CIDI). Weinheim, Beltz Test, 1990.
18 Dilling H, Mombour W, Schmidt MH (eds): Internationale Klassifikation psychischer Störungen. ICD-10 Kapitel V (F). Bern, Huber, 1993.
19 Buchsbaum MS, Silverman J: Stimulus intensity control and the cortical evoked response. Psychosom Med 1968;30:12–22.
20 Connolly, JF, Gruzelier, JH: Amplitude and latency changes in the visual evoked potential to different stimulus intensities. Psychophysiology 1982;19:599–608.
21 Carton S, Jouvent R, Bungener C, Widlöcher D: Sensation seeking and depressive mood. Pers Individ Diff 1992;13:843–849.

Neuropsychobiology

Neuropsychobiology 2000;41:31–37

Is Resting Anterior EEG Alpha Asymmetry a Trait Marker for Depression?

Findings for Healthy Adults and Clinically Depressed Patients

Stefan Debener[a] André Beauducel[a] Doreen Nessler[a,b] Burkhard Brocke[a] Hubert Heilemann[c] Jürgen Kayser[d]

[a]Department of Psychology II, Dresden University of Technology, Dresden, [b]Max Planck Institute of Cognitive Neuroscience, Leipzig, [c]State Mental Hospital Arnsdorf, Germany, and [d]Department of Biopsychology, New York State Psychiatric Institute, New York, N.Y., USA

Key Words
Depression · Emotion · Laterality · Anterior brain activation · EEG alpha power · Resting EEG · Temporal stability

Abstract
Several lines of evidence suggest that asymmetric anterior brain activation is related to affective style, linking left hemisphere activation to positive affect and right hemisphere activation to negative affect. However, previous reports of left frontal hypoactivation in depressed patients were not confirmed in recent studies. This study evaluated additional characteristics of resting EEG alpha (8–13 Hz) asymmetry in 15 clinically depressed patients and 22 healthy adults by recording EEG activity on two separate occasions, 2–4 weeks apart. Across both sessions, group differences in anterior EEG asymmetry were compatible with the original hypothesis. However, groups differed in temporal stability of anterior EEG asymmetry, which was retest reliable in controls but not depressed patients. In contrast, temporal stability of posterior EEG asymmetry was acceptable in both groups. Increased variability of anterior EEG asymmetry may be a characteristic feature for depression, and, if so, this would challenge the notion that anterior EEG alpha asymmetry is a trait marker for depression.

Introduction

A growing body of evidence strongly suggests that the right and left cerebral hemispheres are differentially involved in the regulation and processing of emotion [1]. During the past two decades, anterior electroencephalographic (EEG) alpha power asymmetry, an inverse measure of relative brain activation, has been related to hemispheric specialization of fundamental dimensions of affect, resulting in a model of anterior asymmetry and emotion [1, 2]. This model postulates an association between individual differences in anterior activation asymmetry and emotion: individuals with a relative stronger left-sided activation are biased toward positive-valenced stimuli and approach-related behavior, whereas those with a relative stronger right-sided activation are biased to negative-valenced stimuli and withdrawal-related behavior. In agreement with this hypothesis is that brain-damaged patients with lesions in left frontal areas also showed symptoms of depression [3, but see also 4]. Because temperament abnormalities in depression are commonly characterized by low positive emotionality, i.e. loss of pleasurable engagement [5], reduced left anterior activation may be related to core symptoms of depression.

Left anterior hypoactivation during rest, as reflected by increased left frontal EEG power in the alpha band (8–13 Hz), has been reported in acute depressed [6] as well as

KARGER
Fax + 41 61 306 12 34
E-Mail karger@karger.ch
www.karger.com

0302–282X/00/0411–0031$17.50/0

Accessible online at:
www.karger.com/journals/nps

Stefan Debener, Dipl.-Psych.
TU Dresden, Institut für Psychologie II
Mommsenstrasse 13
D–01062 Dresden (Germany)
E-Mail debener@rcs.urz.tu-dresden.de

remitted patients [7]. In nondepressed individuals, resting EEG alpha asymmetry was found to be stable over time [8–10] and therefore assumed to reflect individual differences. In further agreement with the anterior asymmetry and emotion model is that anterior EEG alpha asymmetry, firstly, predicted affective reactivity [11] and, secondly, showed a relation to individual differences in temperament [10, 12, 13]. Infant studies emphasize the importance of asymmetric anterior brain activation for behavior that is associated with biological features of depression [1]. Hence, functional anterior brain asymmetry has been considered as trait marker for the vulnerability to depression, and left anterior hypoactivation in depression is hypothesized to reflect underactivation of the approach system [1, 2].

For several years, brain activation has been explored by means of quantitative EEG, where EEG alpha activity (8–13 Hz) is considered as an inverse correlate of cerebral activation [14]. Recent imaging evidence seems to support this assumption. Using positron emission tomography (PET), Cook et al. [15] found a significant negative correlation between absolute power in the EEG alpha frequency range and simultaneously recorded $H^{15}{}_2O$ PET-derived cortical activation [15].

Subclinically depressed college students identified by high scores on the Beck depression inventory (BDI) showed increased left frontal alpha power, which is interpreted as left frontal hypoactivation [16]. Similar relations of BDI scores to anterior EEG asymmetry were also reported for healthy men [13]. Among clinically depressed patients, there is ample evidence of left-sided [17] or left anterior hypoactivation [6, 18–21], although there are also several contradictory findings [22–24]. However, studies differ widely in EEG methodology (e.g. recording and epoch length, site of reference electrode), patient diagnosis and symptomatology, and medication status. At least, these methodological differences cause tremendous problems when comparing findings. For example, the internal consistency of EEG alpha power asymmetry is inadequate when based on 1-min recording intervals [25]. As another problem, the studies cited above differ with respect to the particular anterior scalp locations (F3/4, F7/8, T3/4) and the specific recording condition (eyes open vs. eyes closed) for which significant effects were found.

From a theoretical point, empirical evidence according to the hypothesized state independence of left frontal hypoactivation in depression is important, particularly because mood states are suspected to modify resting anterior alpha asymmetry in depression [26]. Only one clinical study reported EEG findings for depressed patients that were repeatedly tested [27]. In this study, left anterior hypoactivation was unchanged in patients with seasonal affective disorder (SAD) after 2 weeks of phototherapy. However, the study's results are based on a small sample size of four, and a generalization from SAD to other depressive subtypes is questionable. Therefore, the study by Allen et al. [27] does not provide an adequate estimate for the temporal stability of anterior asymmetry in depression.

The present study aimed to investigate the temporal stability of anterior EEG alpha power asymmetry in a larger sample of depressed patients and healthy adults. Based on the majority of findings reported in the literature, we hypothesized that left anterior hypoactivation, as indicated by greater left than right alpha power in resting EEG, will be related to depression. Furthermore, anterior EEG asymmetry was predicted to serve as trait index of depression and should consequently be stable over time in both clinically depressed patients and healthy adults.

Method

Participants

Depressed inpatients were recruited from the depression ward of the State Mental Hospital Arnsdorf, Germany, so that participation did not affect therapeutic treatment. Diagnosis and clinical state were assessed on separate sessions within a few days of the EEG recording sessions. A structural clinical interview [28] was taken by a trained graduate student, and consensus diagnosis was established together with an experienced psychiatrist (H.H.). Patients were excluded if they had a past history or current symptoms of bipolar affective disorder, organic brain disorder, psychosis or substance abuse. Patients were also excluded if there was a change in medication status during the time of participation, since means of treatment were unaffected by participation in this study.

Patients who received lithium as medication were removed from further analysis, because lithium is known to modify EEG alpha asymmetry [29, 30]. Whether other psychotropic medication systematically alters frontal EEG alpha asymmetry is not known yet. In one study on rhesus monkeys [31], diazepam caused a decrease in power in the 4- to 8-Hz frequency band, most pronounced in the left frontal region. In humans, alterations in EEG alpha asymmetry due to antidepressants were not evident [32, 33], nor did experimental variations of serotonergic activity alter EEG alpha asymmetry [34], but this evidence is based on only a few relevant studies. Although several pharmaco-EEG studies analyzed effects of antidepressants, data analysis was typically restricted to midline positions [35]. Therefore, these studies do not provide topographic information. In one recent drug study, the therapeutic effects of the two antidepressants tianeptine and fluvoxamine were associated with a shift in anterior EEG alpha power asymmetry [36] in healthy individuals. As of yet, it is unclear whether psychotropic antidepressants have a normalizing effect with regard to brain activation asymmetry, as assessed by EEG alpha power. Further research is necessary to address this issue.

From the initial sample of 33 retested patients within the course of this study, 18 patients had to be excluded after all clinical information became available after testing. This report includes only those 15 patients who met all inclusion criteria. According to the International Classification of Diseases [37], 2 patients were diagnosed as having a medium depressive episode (F32.1), and 13 patients had a severe depressive episode without psychotic symptoms (F32.2), 1 of them also meeting criteria for dysthymia (F34.1). The majority of patients were initially tested after receiving a fixed dosage of psychotropic antidepressant medication for at least 6 days, with most patients being on fixed dosage for a considerably longer period. Patients received trimipramine (n = 8), doxepin (n = 3), amitriptyline (n = 2), or citalopram (n = 1). Eleven patients received additional anxiolytic medication (lorazepam). One patient did not receive any psychotropic medication. Hospital staff and interested volunteers were recruited as controls through locally posted advertisements, and screened for current or past history of psychiatric illness or substance abuse. A retest for all participants was scheduled 2–4 weeks after the initial EEG recording session. Handedness was assessed with the Edinburgh Handedness Inventory [38]. Participants were also requested to report their mood on the BDI [39], and the Positive and Negative Affect Scales [40] were assessed immediately after EEG data collection. Demographic and self-report data for both patient and control groups are summarized in table 1. Among the patients were 10 females and 5 males, the control group consisted of a similar gender ratio of 15 females and 7 males. Although control participants were not selected to match the patients in gender, age, education and handedness, sample characteristics were kept similar to facilitate group comparisons. Whereas group differences in resting EEG alpha power asymmetry are not well known for gender, handedness is suspected to covary with resting brain activation asymmetry [41]. Written informed consent was obtained from all participants.

Table 1. Demographic and self-report data

	Patients (n = 15)	Controls (n = 22)
Gender, women:men	10:5	15:7
Age, mean (range)	48.5 (23–64)	45.9 (26–64)
Education, mean ± SD	9.4 ± 1.6[1]	9.7 ± 1.9
Handedness, left:right	1:14	3:19
Days between EEG recording sessions, mean ± SD	22.5 ± 4.7	21.7 ± 4.2
BDI[2], mean ± SD	20.8 ± 11.2[3]	5.1 ± 3.7
State mood, session 1		
Positive affect, mean ± SD	2.7 ± 0.9	2.9 ± 0.8
Negative affect, mean ± SD	1.5 ± 0.5	1.1 ± 0.2
State mood, session 2		
Positive affect, mean ± SD	2.7 ± 0.8[1]	3.0 ± 0.6
Negative affect, mean ± SD	1.5 ± 0.5[1]	1.1 ± 0.2

1 n = 14.
2 Groups differed significantly, $t_{(12.3)} = 4.8$, $p < 0.001$ (two tailed).
3 n = 12.

EEG Data Collection and Quantification

EEG data were collected from 19 scalp positions during four 2-min periods while participants were resting quietly in a comfortable armchair. Each period of resting EEG was recorded with either eyes open (O) or eyes closed (C). Order of conditions was the same in both EEG sessions, and counterbalanced across participants (i.e. OCOC or COCO).

A Ceegraph AC amplifier system and a stretch lycra cap were used to collect EEG data from 19 scalp locations (10-20 system). Using a forehead ground and linked earlobes (A1-A2) as reference, recordings were taken from 3 midline sites (Fz, Cz, Pz) and 8 homologous pairs of electrodes over each hemisphere (Fp1/2, F3/4, F7/8, C3/4, T3/4, T5/6, P3/4, O1/2). EEG impedances were kept below 5,000 Ω and within 500 Ω at homologous sites, including A1-A2. Vertical electro-oculograms were recorded to facilitate artifact recognition. The EEG signal was band-pass filtered (0.1–30 Hz) and digitized at 256 Hz. Continuous EEG data were divided offline in 2-second epochs (75% overlap) and rejected if visual inspection indicated eye movements or other recording artifacts. For eyes open, controls produced more artifact-free epochs than patients across recording sessions (controls, mean = 258, range 71–400, vs. patients, mean = 137, range 41–321; $t_{(35)} = 4.02$, $p < 0.001$), but there were no group differences for eyes closed (controls, mean = 326, range 77–458, vs. patients, mean = 350, range 153–462; $t_{(35)} = -0.70$, n.s.). However, as stated below, internal consistency of EEG alpha power asymmety was highly reliable across conditions in both groups. A Hamming window [9] was then applied over the distal 50% of each epoch. Absolute spectral power (μV^2) as a function of frequency was derived by means of fast Fourier transformation. Epochs were averaged separately for eyes open and eyes closed condition. Power density values were then ln transformed to normalize data [42]. Statistical analyses were restricted to power in the EEG alpha band (8–13 Hz) to limit Type I error probability, and because previous studies on individual differences in anterior activation asymmetry have focused on this frequency range.

Statistical Analysis

Previous studies involving measures of anterior asymmetry have reported effects at mid-frontal (F3/4), lateral-frontal (F7/8), and anterior-temporal (T3/4) sites (see [24] for a detailed discussion). For these locations, significant parametric intercorrelations of asymmetry measures were obtained in the present data for depressed patients (r = 0.68–0.94) and healthy controls (r = 0.69–0.94). Therefore, electrode sites were pooled within anterior left (F3, F7, T3) and right (F4, F8, T4) regions to reduce the amount of data [17]. Like previous studies, mid-parietal (P3, P4) sites were included to control for regional effects of EEG alpha power [7, 16].

To examine the hypothesized group differences in anterior alpha asymmetry, data from the two recording sessions were submitted to a 2 × 2 × 2 × 2 repeated-measures analysis of variance (ANOVA), including session (1, 2), hemisphere (left, right), and region (anterior, posterior) as within-subjects factors, and group (patients, controls) as a between-subjects factor. Significant interactions were examined through simple effects to locate the source of interaction (BMDP-4V) [43]. To increase statistical power, condition (eyes open, eyes closed) was not included as factor. Furthermore, an explicit goal of this study was to evaluate psychometric properties of alpha asymmetry for both groups separately, and, as described below, this evaluation involved both recording conditions.

Asymmetry measures were also computed by subtracting left-sided power density from right-sided power density at homologous sites (ln right minus ln left). Higher scores on this asymmetry index are interpreted to reflect greater left-sided activation [10]. Temporal stability (rest-retest reliability) of alpha power asymmetry was examined by

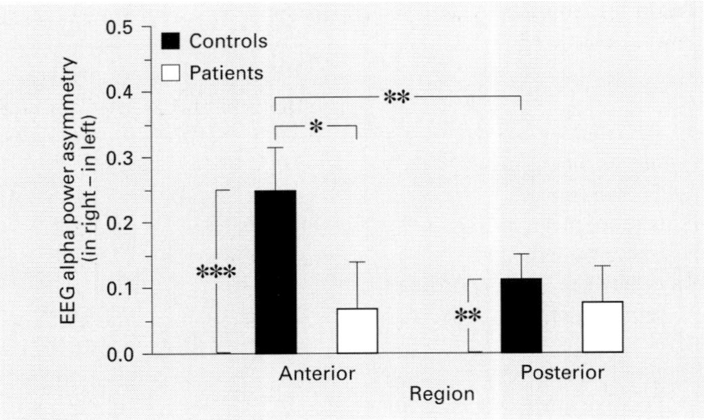

Fig. 1. Mean (± SEM) alpha asymmetry (ln right minus ln left) scores at anterior and posterior sites for healthy controls and depressed patients, averaged over session 1 and session 2. Positive scores indicate more left hemispheric activation. Means were collapsed across mid-frontal (F3, F4), lateral-frontal (F7, F8) and anterior-temporal (T3, T4) sites for the anterior region, and computed for mid-parietal (P3, P4) sites for the posterior region. The interaction region by group, calculated for the asymmetry indices, was significant, $F(1, 35) = 4.99$, $p = 0.032$. Significant mean differences (simple effects, two tailed) are indicated. *$p < 0.1$; **$p < 0.01$; ***$p < 0.001$.

computing the Pearson correlations separately for the four indices (anterior: F8-F7, F4-F3, T4-T3; posterior: P4-P3). Internal consistency was determined by Cronbach's α computations of alpha power asymmetry indices, based on two measures for eyes open and two measures for eyes closed conditions. These calculations were done separately for each of the four scalp sites of interest and for each of the two recording sessions. To explore the relationship of anterior asymmetry and mood, correlations of positive affect, negative affect, and overall mood [10] to anterior asymmetry measures were performed.

Results

The results of the repeated measures ANOVA revealed significant main effects for group, $F(1, 35) = 5.49$, $p = 0.02$, hemisphere, $F(1, 35) = 11.02$, $p = 0.002$, region, $F(1, 35) = 143.75$, $p < 0.001$, and session, $F(1, 35) = 5.84$, $p = 0.02$. Confirming earlier findings [22], depressed patients (mean = 0.55, SD = 1.05) had more alpha power than nondepressed controls (mean = –0.15, SD = 0.97). As expected, posterior sites (mean = 0.53, SD = 1.09) showed more alpha power than anterior sites (mean = –0.27, SD = 0.86). There was also more alpha power over the right (mean = 0.20, SD = 1.05) than left (mean = 0.06, SD = 1.07) hemisphere, and at session 2 (mean = 0.18, SD = 1.08) than at session 1 (mean = 0.08, SD = 1.04).

A significant hemisphere by region interaction, $F(1, 35) = 4.10$, $p = 0.05$, was indicative of a slightly more pronounced anterior than posterior right-larger-than-left EEG alpha power asymmetry, although simple effects for hemisphere were highly significant for both regions (anterior, $F(1, 35) = 10.52$, $p = 0.003$; posterior, $F(1, 35) = 8.73$, $p = 0.006$). More importantly, there were regionally dependent differences between groups in left-versus right-sided alpha power, which was supported by a significant hemisphere by region by group interaction, $F(1, 35) = 4.99$, $p < 0.032$. Simple interaction effects revealed that the hemisphere by region interaction was significant only for controls, $F(1, 35) = 11.19$, $p = 0.002$, but not for patients, $F(1, 35) = 0.02$, n.s. A suggested hemisphere by group simple interaction effect emerged only at anterior, $F(1, 35) = 3.40$, $p = 0.07$, but not at posterior sites, $F(1, 35) = 0.35$, n.s. Finally, simple hemisphere main effects, calculated for each group and each region, revealed significant greater right than left alpha power only for controls, particularly at anterior sites [anterior, $F(1, 35) = 15.96$, $p < 0.001$; posterior, $F(1, 35) = 7.76$, $p = 0.009$], but not for patients [anterior, $F(1, 35) = 0.82$, n.s.; posterior, $F(1, 35) = 2.34$, n.s.). No other significant interaction effects were found in the overall $2 \times 2 \times 2 \times 2$ analysis.

To illustrate the interaction effects involving hemisphere, EEG alpha power asymmetries (ln right minus ln left) are plotted in figure 1 (interaction effects of two-level factors are statistically equivalent to lower-order effects in an ANOVA on level difference scores). Collapsed across both sessions, controls showed a pronounced left sided activation over the anterior region, i.e. more right than left hemisphere alpha power, and less pronounced left-sided activation over posterior sites, whereas EEG alpha power asymmetry was insignificant in patients for both regions. In contrast to EEG alpha power asymmetry over anterior regions, posterior asymmetry did not differ significantly between patients and controls.

To facilitate comparison with previous research, and because a session main effect indicated overall differences in EEG alpha power between both testing sessions, repeated-measures ANOVA were computed post hoc for each session. These analyses revealed for session 1 suggestive interactions of hemisphere by group, $F(1, 35) = 3.56$, $p = 0.07$, and hemisphere by region by group, $F(1, 35) = 3.23$, $p = 0.08$. In session 2, neither of these interactions reached statistical significance [hemisphere by group, $F(1, 35) = 0.50$, n.s.; hemisphere by region by group, $F(1, 35) = 2.31$, $p = 0.14$].[1]

[1] To address the concern that variations in vigilance may affect group differences in EEG alpha asymmetry, data were reanalyzed by including a factor *vigilance*, which was operationalized by comparing the first 4 min and the last 4 min of each 8-min recording session. Neither the corresponding five-way

We further examined internal consistency and temporal stability for each group. Internal consistency computations for each of the four homologous electrode pairs were based on four asymmetry measures during rest, i.e. two measures with eyes open, and two measures with eyes closed. Internal consistencies ranged from 0.84 to 0.98 in the control group, and from 0.87 to 0.98 in the patient group (table 2). These results strongly suggest that EEG alpha power provides a reliable asymmetry measure, irrespective of group, region and session, when averaged over condition (eyes open vs. eyes closed). Excellent reliability in both groups further indicated that group differences in the number of artifact-free epochs (see above) did not bear on reliability.

For nondepressed individuals, temporal stability of EEG alpha power asymmetry (table 2) revealed significant stabilities across the different scalp regions (r = 0.46–0.69). For depressed patients, however, a significant test-retest stability of r = 0.57 emerged only for mid-parietal sites; for anterior regions, correlations between recording sessions 2–4 weeks apart were around zero (r = –0.22 to 0.09) and not significant.

Additional correlational analyses of self-reported positive and negative affect scores did not reveal any systematic relationship to EEG alpha power asymmetry, neither in patients nor in controls.

Table 2. Internal consistency and temporal stability of EEG alpha power asymmetry

	Internal consistency session 1/session 2	Temporal stability
Patients (n = 15)		
Mid-frontal	0.87/0.94	0.09
Lateral-frontal	0.96/0.98	–0.22
Anterior-temporal	0.97/0.98	–0.05
Mid-parietal	0.95/0.91	0.57*
Controls (n = 22)		
Mid-frontal	0.94/0.95	0.69**
Lateral-frontal	0.97/0.98	0.46*
Anterior-temporal	0.93/0.97	0.53*
Mid-parietal	0.84/0.95	0.68**

Internal consistency based on Cronbach's α, temporal stability estimations computed as Pearson's correlations. *p < 0.05; **p < 0.01 (two tailed).

Discussion

The present study evaluated regional characteristics and their statistical properties of asymmetric brain activation in depression by assessing EEG alpha power during rest at two different recording sessions. In agreement with prior findings [6, 18–21], depressed patients differed from healthy controls in resting anterior EEG asymmetry when data were collapsed across the two recording sessions separated by 2–4 weeks. Depressed patients failed to show more left than right anterior alpha activity, whereas healthy controls had markedly more right than left anterior alpha activity, i.e. a relative greater activation of left anterior regions. No group differences were found for mid-parietal EEG asymmetry. Although it should clearly be noted that the lack of frontal EEG asymmetry seen in depressed patients did not exactly match previous findings, the direction of group differences in frontal EEG asymmetry is in line with the theory of a left frontal hypoactivation in depression.

In our study, anterior EEG asymmetry was based on alpha power collapsed across three anterior sites (F3/4, F7/8, T3/4), since initial data analyses did not show any systematic differences in EEG asymmetry for these locations. Furthermore, internal consistency measures of EEG alpha power asymmetry revealed excellent scores of Cronbach's α for both patients and controls, regardless of scalp region. This finding extends previous research of EEG alpha power asymmetry in healthy individuals [8, 9, 25], by demonstrating that this measure is similarly reliable in clinically depressed patients.

In the present study, EEG alpha asymmetry was solely calculated on the basis of data derived by a linked-earlobes reference, although this reference is critically discussed in the literature [44]. In a previous study [45], we compared linked-earlobes-referenced data to computational Cz-referenced and common-average-referenced data (19-channel recording). The linked-earlobes reference channel comprised less alpha activity in a resting condition, and the corresponding data reflected more appropriately the basic occipitoparietal topography of EEG alpha activity in healthy individuals. However, the results in this report should be interpreted minding the linked earlobes reference, because asymmetry measures derived by different ways of EEG reference may [6, 7, 9, 11] or may not [24, 25, 45] provide similar results. Future work should address this issue with high-density EEG

ANOVA hemisphere × region × session × vigilance × group nor calculations done separately for each recording session revealed evidence for a significant contribution of the factor vigilance (i.e. for the main effect of vigilance and all interactions involving vigilance, p > 0.10).

recordings to provide higher spatial resolution and the possibility for several additional reference montages.

More importantly, group differences emerged for the analysis of temporal characteristics in anterior EEG asymmetry. Whereas posterior EEG asymmetry was acceptably stable over time in both patients and controls, only controls showed adequate temporal stability of anterior EEG asymmetry. For controls, the level of test-retest stability confirms earlier reports [8–10]. Concerning the insufficient stability of anterior EEG asymmetry in depressed patients, our results differ clearly from one previous report that investigated only four bipolar patients [27]. The group differences in temporal stability of anterior EEG alpha power asymmetry reported here were not biased due to group differences in reliability (internal consistency). It is therefore likely that the temporal instability of anterior EEG alpha power asymmetry provides essential, additional information when characterizing depressed patients in terms of EEG correlates.

Our finding of instable anterior EEG alpha power asymmetry in patients is particularly noteworthy, because this measure has been considered a trait marker for depression [7]. Several reasons may contribute to this instability. First, there is preliminary evidence on an association of state affect and EEG alpha power asymmetry in depression [26]. For this reason, we have explored the relation of the subjects' self-reported mood and anterior EEG asymmetry, but neither in healthy controls nor in depressed patients did we find a significant relation between positive affect, negative affect or a combined measure of mood and anterior EEG asymmetry [for methodology, 10]. Thus, we did not find evidence that state mood is linked to variations in frontal EEG asymmetry, but, of course, we cannot exclude this possibility.

Second, the majority of depressed patients received pharmacological treatment during the course of the study. Although antidepressants are generally not known to alter EEG alpha asymmetry [32, 33], a few studies have related therapeutic effects of antidepressants to a shift in anterior EEG alpha power asymmetry [29, 36]. As stated in the Method section, patients were only included in the study if their medication did not change between testing sessions. However, since patient medication was determined by the course of clinical treatment rather than by the experimental design, the possible influence of antidepressants on anterior EEG alpha asymmetry and its temporal characteristics was uncontrolled in this study. Whether regionally restricted alteration of anterior EEG asymmetry is caused by antidepressant medication is not known yet. Future research may determine whether mood improvements in clinically depressed patients due to antidepressant medication are accompanied by a shift towards higher left anterior activation.

A third reason for the observed instabile anterior EEG asymmetry in depressed patients may derive from the fact that other clinical symptoms, which often accompany mood disorders, but do not represent core symptoms of depression, could also have an impact on asymmetric brain activation. In particular, different forms of anxiety are associated with different patterns of asymmetric hemispheric activation, thereby raising the issue that a comorbidity of depression and anxiety may conversely affect EEG topography [17, 46]. It is conceivable, that different clinical symptoms obscure EEG lateralities and vary over time. However, it was beyond the scope of this study to investigate the influence of possible mediator variables like different forms of anxiety.

The temporal instability of anterior EEG alpha power asymmetry in depressed patients is also most likely the cause for the weak relationship of anterior EEG asymmetry to depression that was found in separate analyses for each recording session. If increased variability of anterior EEG asymmetry is indeed a characteristic feature for depression in general, or for some depressive subtypes, this fact may then help to explain recent failures to replicate earlier reports on left frontal hypoactivation in depression. Most previous studies collected EEG data simply only at *one* recording session [6, 16–21, 23; for a discussion on further possibilities for these failures, see 24]. Although our findings clearly need independent replication, a major goal for future studies should be to unveil circumstances that lead to temporal instability of asymmetric EEG activation seen over anterior brain regions.

To sum up, the findings reported in this study add to the growing body of evidence to show alterations of anterior brain activation in depression. Since anterior EEG asymmetry lacked temporal stability in depressed patients in this study, it appears too premature to consider anterior EEG alpha power asymmetry a trait marker for depression. Further research is needed to uncover the temporal characteristics of anterior EEG asymmetry to clinical features of depression.

Acknowledgments

We are grateful to R. John, A. Naumann, S. Raabe, D. Schulze and the hospital staff for their help. We also acknowledge the technical support of J. Schäfer, G. Pascher and V. Hantzsch, and thank G. Erdmann for discussions that proved useful in writing this article.

References

1 Davidson RJ: Cerebral asymmetry, emotion, and affective style; in Davidson RJ, Hugdahl K (eds): Brain Asymmetry. Cambridge, MIT, 1995, pp 361–387.
2 Davidson RJ: Affective style and affective disorders: Perspectives from affective neuroscience. Cogn Emotion 1998;12:307–330.
3 Robinson RG, Downhill JE: Lateralization of psychopathology in response to focal brain injury; in Davidson RJ, Hugdahl K (eds): Brain Asymmetry. Cambridge, MIT, 1995, pp 693–711.
4 Borod, JC: Interhemispheric and intrahemispheric control of emotion: A focus on unilateral brain damage. J Consult Clin Psychol 1992;60: 339–348.
5 Fowles DC: Psychophysiology and psychopathology: A motivational approach. Psychophysiology 1987;25:373–391.
6 Henriques JB, Davidson RJ: Left frontal hypoactivation in depression. J Abnorm Psychol 1991; 100:22–31.
7 Henriques JB, Davidson RJ: Regional brain electrical asymmetries discriminate between previously depressed and normal control subjects. J Abnorm Psychol 1990;99:22–31.
8 Papousek I, Schulter G: Different temporal stability and partial independence of EEG asymmetries from different locations: Implications for laterality research. Int J Neurosci 1998;93: 87–100.
9 Tomarken AJ, Davidson RJ, Wheeler RE, Kinney L: Psychometric properties of resting anterior EEG asymmetry: Temporal stability and internal consistency. Psychophysiology 1992; 29:576–592.
10 Sutton SK, Davidson RJ: Prefrontal brain asymmetry: A biological substrate of the behavioral approach and inhibition systems. Psychol Sci 1997;8:204–210.
11 Wheeler RE, Davidson RJ, Tomarken AJ: Frontal brain asymmetry and emotional reactivity: A biological substrate of affective style. Psychophysiology 1993;30:82–89.
12 Harmon-Jones E, Allen JJB: Behavioral activation sensitivity and resting frontal EEG asymmetry: Covariation of putative indicators related to risk for mood disorders. J Abnorm Psychol 1997;106:159–163.
13 Jacobs GD, Snyder D: Frontal brain asymmetry predicts affective style in men. Behav Neurosci 1996;110:3–6.
14 Schagass C: Electrical activity in the brain; in Greenfield NS, Sternbach RA (eds): Handbook of Psychophysiology. Hillsdale, Erlbaum, 1972, pp 263–328.
15 Cook IA, O'Hara R, Uijtdehaage SHJ, Mandelkern M, Leuchter AF: Assessing the accuracy of topographic EEG mapping for determining local brain function. Electroencephalogr Clin Neurophysiol 1998;107:408–414.
16 Schaffer CE, Davidson RJ, Sarron C: Frontal and parietal electroencephalogram asymmetry in depressed and nondepressed subjects. Biol Psychiatry 1983;18:753–762.
17 Bruder GE, Fong R, Tenke CE, Leite P, Towey JP, Stewart JE, McGrath PJ, Quitkin FM: Regional brain asymmetries in major depression with or without an anxiety disorder: A quantitative electroencephalographic study. Biol Psychiatry 1997;41:939–948.
18 Kano K, Nakamura M, Matsuoka T, Iida H, Nakajima T: The topographical features of EEGs in patients with affective disorders. Electroencephalogr Clin Neurophysiol 1992;83: 124–129.
19 Roemer RA, Schagass C, Dubin W, Jaffe R, Siegal L: Quantitative EEG in elderly depressives. Brain Topogr 1992;4:285–290.
20 Saletu B, Brandstätter N, Metka M, Stamenkovic M, Anderer P, Semlitsch HV, Heytmanek G, Huber J, Grünberger J, Linzmayer L, Kurz C, Decker K, Binder G, Knogler W, Koll B: Hormonal, syndromal and EEG mapping studies in menopausal syndrome patients with and without depression as compared with controls. Maturitas 1996;23:91–105.
21 Bell IR, Schwartz GE, Hardin EE, Baldwin CM, Kline JP: Differential resting quantitative electroencephalographic alpha patterns in women with environmental chemical intolerance, depressives, and normals. Biol Psychiatry 1998;43:376–388.
22 Pollock VE, Schneider LS: Quantitative, waking EEG research on depression. Biol Psychiatry 1990;27:757–780.
23 Pollock VE, Schneider LS: Topographic quantitative EEG in elderly subjects with major depression. Psychophysiology 1990;27:438–444.
24 Reid SA, Duke LM, Allen JJB: Resting frontal electroencephalographic asymmetry in depression: Inconsistencies suggest the need to identify mediating factors. Psychophysiology 1998; 35:389–404.
25 Hagemann D, Naumann E, Becker G, Maier S, Bartussek D: Frontal brain asymmetry and affective style: A conceptual replication. Psychophysiology 1998;35:372–388.
26 Rosenfeld JP, Baehr E, Baehr R, Gotlib ICH, Ranganath C: Preliminary evidence that daily changes in frontal alpha asymmmetry correlate with changes in affect in therapy sessions. Int J Psychophysiol 1996;23:137–141.
27 Allen JJ, Iacono WG, Depue RA, Arbisi P: Regional EEG asymmetries in bipolar seasonal affective disorder before and after phototherapy. Biol Psychiatry 1993;33:642–646.
28 Pfister H, Wittchen H, Weigel A: Composite International Diagnostic Interview (CIDI). Weinheim, Beltz Test, 1990.
29 Ulrich G, Frick K, Lewinsky M: Lithium and the theoretical concept of 'dynamic restriction': A comparison of the effects on different levels of quantitative EEG analysis. Lithium 1993;4: 33–44.
30 Thau K, Rappelsberger P, Lovrek A, Petsche H, Simhandl C, Topitz A: Effect of lithium on the EEG of healthy males and females. Neuropsychobiology 1988;20:158–163.
31 Davidson RJ, Kalin NH, Shelton SE: Lateralized effects of diazepam on frontal brain electrical asymmetries in rhesus monkeys. Biol Psychiatry 1992;32:438–451.
32 Kwon JS, Youn T, Jung HY: Right hemisphere abnormalities in major depression: Quantitative electroencephalographic findings before and after treatment. J Affective Disord 1996; 40:169–173.
33 Shagass C, Roemer RA, Josiassen RC: Some quantitative EEG findings in unmedicated and medicated depressives. Neuropsychobiology 1988;19:169–175.
34 Knott VJ, Howson AL, Perugini M, Ravindran AV, Young SN: The effect of acute tryptophan depletion and fenfluramine on quantitative EEG and mood in healthy male subjects. Biol Psychiatry, in press.
35 Herrmann WM, Schärer E, Wendt G, Delini-Stula A: Pharmaco-EEG profile of levoprotiline. Pharmacopsychiatry 1991;24:206–213.
36 Saletu B, Grünberger J, Anderer P, Linzmayer L, Zyhlarz G: Comparative pharmacodynamic studies with the novel serotonin uptake-enhancing tianeptine and -inhibiting fluvoxamine utilizing EEG mapping and psychometry. J Neural Transm 1996;103:191–216.
37 Dilling H, Mombour W, Schmidt MH (eds): Internationale Klassifikation psychischer Störungen. ICD-10 Kapitel V (F). Bern, Huber, 1993.
38 Oldfield RC: The assessment and analysis of handedness: The Edinburgh inventory. Neuropsychologia 1971;9:97–112.
39 Hautzinger M, Bailer M, Worall H, Keller F: Beck-Depressions-Inventar (BDI), ed 2, rev. Bern, Huber, 1995.
40 Krohne HW, Egloff B, Kohlmann C, Tausch A: Untersuchungen mit einer deutschsprachigen Version der 'Positive and Negative Affect Schedule' (PANAS). Diagnostica 1996;42: 139–156.
41 Debener S, Nessler D, Friedrich C, Brocke B: Zum Einfluss der Händigkeit auf das Spontan-EEG: Alpha-Asymmetrie und interhemisphärische Kohärenz; in Schröger E, Mecklinger A, Widmann A (eds): Experimentelle Psychologie. 41. Tagung experimentell arbeitender Psychologen. Lengerich, Papst Science Publishers, 1999, p 114.
42 Gasser T, Bächer P, Möcks J: Transformations toward the normal distribution of broad band spectral parameters of the EEG. Electroencephalogr Clin Neurophysiol 1982;53:119–124.
43 Dixon WJ (ed): BMDP Statistical Software Manual: To Accompany the 7.0 Software Release. Berkeley, University of California Press, 1992.
44 Miller GA, Lutzenberger W, Elbert T: The linked-reference issue in EEG and ERP recording. J Psychophysiol 1991;5:273–276.
45 Debener S, Beauducel A, Brocke B, Kayser J: Resting anterior EEG alpha asymmetry and affective style: Effects of electrode location and reference (abstract). J Psychophysiol, in press.
46 Heller W, Nitschke JB, Etienne MA, Miller GA: Patterns of regional brain activity differentiate types of anxiety. J Abnorm Psychol 1997;106:376–385.

Neuropsychobiology

Neuropsychobiology 2000;41:38–47

Endocrine Responses after *d*-Fenfluramine and Ipsapirone Challenge: Further Support for Cloninger's Tridimensional Model of Personality

J. Hennig C. Toll P. Schonlau S. Rohrmann P. Netter

Department of Psychology, University of Giessen, Germany

Key Words

d-Fenfluramine · Ipsapirone · Cortisol · Prolactin · Personality

Abstract

The tridemensional model of personality introduced by Cloninger relates aspects of novelty seeking to the dopaminergic, harm avoidance (HA) to the serotonergic, and reward dependence to the noradrenergic neurotransmitter system. Using a neuroendocrine challenge paradigm, this study investigates whether subjects characterized by blunted cortisol (CORT) responses after ipsapirone (IPS) relate to different subfactors of HA from those characterized by blunted prolactin (PRL) responses after treatment with *d*-fenfluramine (D-FEN). Moreover, subjects blunted in both responses should differ in scale values of subfactors of HA from those with only one or no blunted reactions. In the first part of the experiment, 16 healthy male volunteers were treated with 15 mg D-FEN. The second part of the study (about 1 year later) consists of a challenge with the partial 5-hydroxytryptamine-1a (5-HT_{1a}) agonist IPS (10 mg) in the same subjects. The results indicate that blunted PRL responses are accompanied by high values in HA, while the main effect of IPS responsivity did not relate significantly to this dimension. With respect to the subscales of HA, subjects blunted in both responses (PRL–/C–) exhibit significantly higher levels in fatigability and asthenia when compared to all other groups (PRL–/C+, PRL+/C–,PRL+/C+). The data demonstrate that combined challenge tests may shed more light on the biological basis of personality and that HA and most clearly fatigability and asthenia relate to the 5-HT system.

Introduction

Several attempts have been published to investigate functional aspects of the neurotransmitter system 5-hydroxytryptamine (5-HT). Since levels of 5-HT in the cerebrospinal fluid (CSF) have been shown to be extremly low and not very reliable [1], levels of the metabolite 5-hydroxy-indole-acetic-acid (5-HIAA) were chosen as the preferred parameter. However, the observation that tryptophan-rich diet leads to marked changes in levels of 5-HIAA without any changes in the firing rate of the neurons in the raphé nuclei [2] limited the value of 5-HIAA as a direct indicator of 5-HT function. Moreover, since CSF cannot be obtained without a medical indication in healthy volunteers, other indicators should be considered

KARGER

Fax + 41 61 306 12 34
E-Mail karger@karger.ch
www.karger.com

0302–282X/00/0411–0038$17.50/0

Accessible online at:
www.karger.com/journals/nps

Jürgen Hennig, PhD
Department of Psychology, Center for Psychobiology and Behavioral Medicine
University of Giessen, Otto-Behaghel-Strasse 10, D–35394 Giessen (Germany)
Tel. +49 641 99 26 154, Fax +49 641 99 26 159
E-Mail juergen.hennig@psychol.uni-giessen.de

Platelets have been demonstrated to reflect some aspects of central 5-HT characteristics. For example, uptake mechanism, storage and release are comparable to brain mechanisms but 5-HT synthesis does not take place in platelets [3]. However, platelets are valuable for investigating imipramine binding sites, 5-HT_2 receptor characteristics [4] or uptake mechanisms, since the reduction of 5-HT uptake in platelets induced by selective serotonin reuptake inhibitors is correlated with clinical improvement [5]. The monoamineoxidase B (MAO-B) which is also present in platelets has frequently been discussed as being related to 5-HT functions in the CNS, but because of several problems including measurement, the presence of different subpopulations of platelets with different MAO acitvities, and – most importantly – low specificity for diagnostic purposes (low activity in schizophrenics and depressives), other peripheral indicators became necessary [3].

Since changes in 5-HT neurotransmitter levels or activity reliably induce hormone responses, this led to the use of neurotransmitter challenge tests [6–8]. In these, precursors [9, 10], agonists [11] or releasers [12] were investigated with respect to changes in the concentrations of pituitary hormones: growth hormone, adrenocorticotropic hormone (ACTH), prolactin (PRL) or adrenocortical hormones like cortisol (CORT). The basic idea is that the amount of change in hormone concentrations reflects the reactivity of the neurotransmitter system which can be related to clinical states like depression [13–20], impulsive aggression [21–23], obsessive-compulsive disorders [24, 25] and other psychiatric diseases. However, studies relating 5-HT-induced endocrine responses to personality traits are rare. However, an extrapolation from clinical states to personality traits with respect to 5-HT has been demonstrated in the past by other indicators of central 5-HT function like platelet MAO-B [26–28] or CSF 5-HIAA levels [29, 30].

One of the most intensively studied substances used in challenge paradigms is the 5-HT reuptake inhibitor/releaser fenfluramine. Ten years ago, Coccaro [21] stated that aggressive behavior is accompanied by blunted PRL increases after treatment with fenfluramine indicating an overall reduced 5-HT activity. However, this study aimed at investigating a personality *disorder* with a history of aggression, impulsivity, and suicide in the past. Interestingly, in this early publication, a negative correlation between peak PRL responses and impulsivity had been obtained in the group of healthy controls as well. In contrast to this finding, in the same year, Fishbein et al. [31] failed to replicate these findings and, instead, observed higher PRL responses in (drug-free) substance users differing in levels of aggression and/or impulsivity. This finding, however, could not be replicated. So, taken together, there is evidence that serotonergic subsensitivity as indicated by blunted PRL responses is indeed associated with serveral different psychiatric disorders. This subsensitivity has also been claimed to be associated with mania [32, 33] and depression [34–36]. For a more comprehensive review see Newman at al. [37].

Another line of research aimed at investigating a possible receptor specificity for hormone changes on the one hand and psychiatric disorder in particular with respect to depression on the other. This led to the development of (partial) 5-HT_{1a} agonists like flesinoxan, buspirone or ipsapirone (IPS). After treatment with flesinoxan, CORT as well as thermoregulatory responses were significantly different between depressed patients with a history of suicide as compared to those without suicidal behavior, whereas both responses were not correlated with measures of irritability or assault [38]. For buspirone it was shown that the responses of PRL and CORT were not different between major depressives and healthy controls or between melancholic and nonmelancholic patients. However, a main effect for gender could be demonstrated as indicated by higher responses in women than in men [39].

IPS caused increases in CORT and decreases in body core temperature more clearly than changes in PRL [40]. CORT increases after IPS were demonstrated to be blunted in major depression while the hypothermic response was not [41]. Impaired ACTH and CORT responses could be demonstrated for unipolar depression as well [42]. However, others pointed out that the severity of depression must be taken into account, since a positive correlation between severity of disease and hypothermic responses after IPS could be demonstrated [43]. In patients with panic disorder, neuroendocrine and thermoregulatory responses to IPS were attenuated probably reflecting a subsensitivity of pre- and postsynaptic 5-HT_{1a} receptors, but obsessive-compulsive patients did not differ from controls in neuroendocrine or thermoregulatory responses after treatment with IPS [44].

Up to now, there is only one study investigating hormonal changes after treatment with *d*-fenfluramine (D-FEN) and IPS in the same subjects [45]. In 8 subjects with personality disorder PRL responses after D-FEN and CORT responses after IPS were inversely related to ratings of assaultiveness, and hypothermic responses after IPS were correlated with aggression. The two endocrine responses were not related to each other indicating the usefulness of a combined challenge paradigm.

Although most of the studies using challenge tests include healthy controls, little is known about 5-HT challenge tests and altered endocrine responses with respect to personality. However, aggressiveness within the range of normal personality has been shown to be negatively related to D-FEN induced CORT responses in male but not in female subjects. Moreover, PRL was not related to personality independently of gender [46]. In a previous study of our group it could be shown that CORT responses after IPS were reduced in experience seekers and in subjects high on disinhibition [47]. Furthermore, high aggression was associated with blunted PRL responses after D-FEN, but with high CORT responses after IPS in two independent studies [48].

The biosocial theory of personality developed by Cloninger [49] is based on the assumption that the principal neurotransmitter systems dopamine, 5-HT and norepinephrine are related to the corresponding fundamental dimensions of personality: novelty seeking (NS), harm avoidance (HA) and reward dependence (RD). Based on this theory, NS and RD are related to other than serotonergic mechanisms and HA should be associated with high levels of 5-HT. Only few data are available relating HA, a dimension related to insecurity and anxiety, to biological indices of serotonin function. For example, B_{max} values of ^{125}I-lysergic acid diethylamide binding to platelets were significantly and inversely correlated to HA scores [50], whereas platelet imipramine binding was not related to HA in another study [51]. Examination stress has been reported to be associated with higher peripheral levels of 5-HT in subjects scoring high on anxiety [52] and performance was found to be reduced after treatment with fluoxetine in high anxiety subjects [53].

The present study was conducted in order to shed more light into the partly conflicting results relating HA to 5-HT by relating this personality trait (and its facets) to the outcome of neuroendocrine challenge tests in healthy volunteers. Furthermore, it has not yet been demonstrated in healthy subjects, whether endocrine responses after FEN and IPS relate to the same traits. Therefore, we addressed the following questions: (1) are blunted PRL responses after D-FEN and blunted CORT responses after IPS differentially related to different aspects of harm avoidance (i.e. the subscale scores), and (2) are subjects with blunted responses to both drugs (CORT responses to IPS and PRL responses to D-FEN) characterized by subdimensions of HA different from all other possible types of responders?

Methods

Subjects

Sixteen healthy male volunteers between 20 and 35 years participated in this study which consists of two challenge paradigms (D-FEN and IPS). Subjects were nonsmokers, drug free and nonalcoholics. Furthermore, any immunological, endocrine or cardiovascular diseases, signs of acute or chronic infection, past or present psychiatric or psychological interventions led to the exclusion of the proband. All subjects were informed about the study protocol, the drugs applied and their possible side effects. The subjects were allowed to quit the experiment at any time without explanation and gave their written informed consent. The studies were approved by an ethics committee. Subjects were recruited from students of different faculties and received a financial incentive for participating in the study. They were instructed not to take any drugs or caffeine-containing drinks prior to the experiment, to go to bed before midnight, and to eat lunch before 1 p.m. at each session.

FEN Challenge Study

A single oral dose of either 15 mg D-FEN (Isomeride®, Itherapia GmbH, München, Germany) or placebo was administered to the subjects in identical capsules in a randomized balanced crossover design under double-blind conditions at a 1-week interval. Between the two sessions, subjects completed a personality questionnaire (see below). The experiments started at 2 p.m. and began with drawing a first blood sample (baseline). Blood sampling was rendered from an indwelling catheter inserted into the antecubital vein to which the tube was connected invisibly to the subject in an adjacent room. At defined time points (+60, +150, +210, +255 min) further blood samples were collected according to the kinetics and half-life of D-FEN [54]. The blood samples were centrifuged immediately afterwards and serum was pipetted into cups which were kept frozen at –80 °C until they were analyzed. All samples were analyzed for PRL concentrations by a commercial radioimmunoassay test kit (ImmunoChem™ Prolactin, ICN Pharmaceuticals Inc., Costa Mesa, Calif., USA). To avoid additional variance by interassay variation, samples were analyzed within one assay. Serum analysis was carried out blind to the experimental condition.

IPS Challenge Study

Several months later, the same subjects were recruited to participate in the second challenge study. According to a previous study [55] a single dose of 10 mg IPS (Tropon, Bayer, Cologne, Germany) had been administered in a double-blind placebo-controlled crossover design comparable to the method described for the FEN challenge study (FCS). Experiments started at 3 p.m. with a first blood sample (baseline). According to Lesch et al. [56] +35, +55, +90 and +110 min later further blood samples were collected which were centrifuged immediately and frozen until assayed at –80 °C. Also, the CORT analyses of all samples were run in one assay which was obtained by ICN as well.

Personality Assessment

Subjects completed the Tridimensional Personality Questionnaire [57] in a translated German version [58]. This questionnaire consists of three scales (NS, HA and RD), each of which comprises four subscales. The basic assumption of the underlying model is that NS relates to dopamine, HA to 5-HT and RD to norepinephrine. The subscales of NS and RD are of minor importance for the present

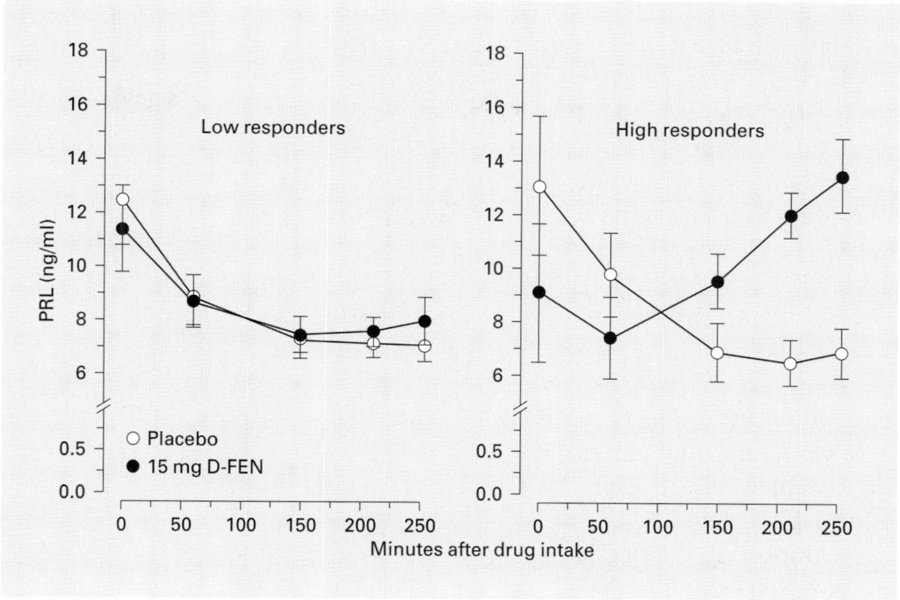

Fig. 1. Means ± SEM of PRL concentrations according to drug (15 mg D-FEN vs. placebo) and response classification by inspection (for statistics see text).

paper since theoretically both substances (D-FEN and IPS) should be related specifically to the 5-HT system. The subscales for HA are: anticipatory worry and pessimism, fear of uncertainty, shyness with strangers, and fatigability and asthenia.

Previous studies of our group based on larger samples sizes yielded satisfying reliabilities (Cronbach's α) for each of the subscales ranging between 0.73 and 0.81. Furthermore, a factor analysis of the four subscales of harm avoidances yielded a single factor explaining 63% of the variance. Correlations between the subscales and the total score of HA were found ranging between 0.74 and 0.82.

Treatment of the Data and Statistical Analysis

Since in both studies (FCS and IPS challenge study) hormone responses could be compared between the drug and the placebo condition within each subject (crossover), a simultaneous visual inspection of response curves could be performed. This procedure was based on several criteria including the comparison of differences between placebo and drug-induced hormone changes, the *probability* of a drug response with respect to the time point of onset (keeping the kinetic of the substance in mind), and – if necessary – an adjustment of baseline values between the placebo and drug session. This procedure resulted in 10 blunted and 6 nonblunted responders in the D-FEN as well as in the IPS part of the study. To validate the effectiveness of this procedure, a discriminant analysis was computed with the responder classification obtained by inspection as group variable and the hormonal profiles as the predicted variables. In both parts of the study (PRL responses after D-FEN and CORT responses after IPS) 14 out of 16 subjects were classified correspondingly. Furthermore, an analysis of variance for repeated measures was computed for substance (repeated measurement factor, drugs vs. placebo), time points (repeated measurement factor, 5 levels) and responder classification as the independent factor to validate the response classification in terms of effect sizes given by eta^2. To evaluate the hypothesis of the specific relation between hormone responses to HA, the three total scores of the dimensions proposed by Cloninger (NS, HA, RD) were subjected to a multivariate analysis of variance with response classification as the independent variable. Since three dimensions were compared, an adjustment of the α-level according to Bonferroni became necessary. The analysis of relationships between hormone responses and subfactors of HA was computed correspondingly with the exception that the level of significance had to be divided by 4.

Results

Since the responder classification was based on visual inspection of the changes under placebo and drug condition, it should be mentioned first that this procedure clearly differentiates subjects with blunted from those with nonblunted hormone responses after challenge with D-FEN or IPS, respectively. The analysis of variance for PRL changes after D-FEN demonstrates that the three-way interaction (drug × responder × time) became highly significant ($F = 5.87$; d.f. = 4, 12; $p < 0.01$) and, furthermore, yielded an effect size explaining about 30% of the total variance ($eta^2 = 0.33$). The time course of hormone changes according to the drug condition and response classification is depicted in figure 1.

Also, the corresponding procedure for IPS-induced changes in CORT reveals a highly significant three-way interaction (drug × responder × time) indicating the validity of the response classification ($F = 8.36$; d.f. = 4, 12; $p < 0.01$). Moreover, the effect size is large and explains more than 75% of the variance ($eta^2 = 0.77$). Drug-

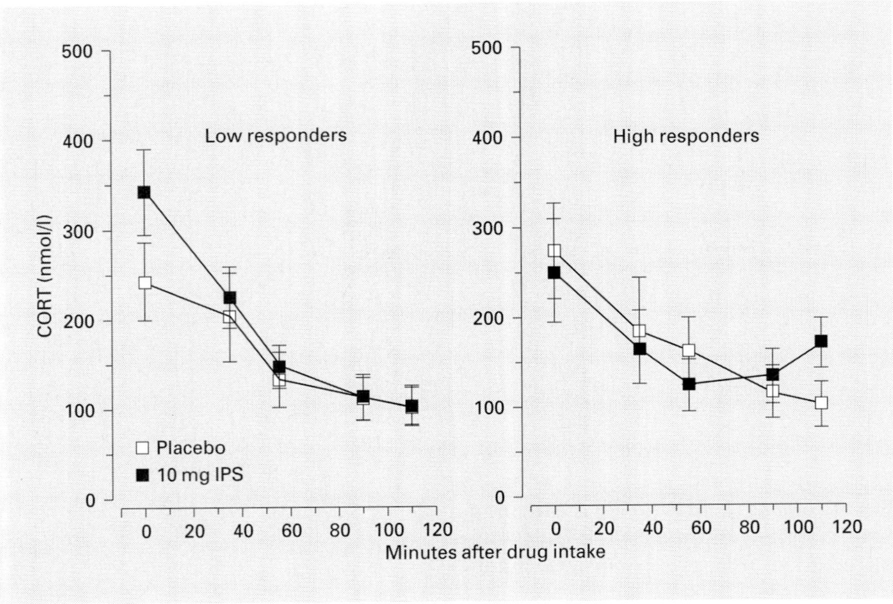

Fig. 2. Means ± SEM of CORT concentrations according to drug (10 mg IPS vs. placebo) and response classification by inspection (for statistics see text).

induced changes in CORT responses according to the response classification are given in figure 2.

As can be clearly seen in figure 2, CORT responses after IPS are generally weak. While hormone responses in subjects exhibiting blunted responses do not differ from the concentrations obtained after placebo, a small increase can be seen in subjects classified as nonblunted. However, although the increase in high responders is low, the effect size is higher than that obtained for PRL responses after D-FEN. This may be due to the nearly identical pattern of changes in CORT after drug and placebo within subjects with blunted responses.

The next hypothesis related to the question if hormone responses after both challenges relate to harm avoidance according to the theory of Cloninger. The multivariate analysis of variance performed for all three principal personality dimensions (NS, HA and RD) demonstrates that PRL responses after D-FEN do not relate to NS ($F = 2.87$; d.f. = 1, 14; p = n.s.) and RD ($F = 0.75$; d.f. = 1, 14; p = n.s.), but only to HA ($F = 6.32$; d.f. = 1, 14; $p < 0.05$). Subjects with blunted responses reveal higher scores in this dimension. However, as described in the methods section, a consequent adjustment of the α-level (according to Bonferroni, 0.05/3 = 0.016) must lead to the conclusion that the effect described did not reveal statistical significance. For CORT changes after IPS, no relationship between the size of responses and the three major personality factors could be found (NS: $F = 0.27$, d.f. = 1, 14, p = n.s.; HA: $F = 0.84$, d.f. = 1, 14, p = n.s.; RD: $F = 0.01$, d.f. = 1, 14, p = n.s.). Means and standard errors for personality dimensions according to the classification of responses in both studies are given in figure 3.

The next question relates to primary factors (= subscales) of HA. Taken together, after adjustment of the α-level (0.05/4 = 0.0125) none of the comparisons in either study became significant. However, there was a tendency of a relation of blunted PRL responses to fatigability and asthenia ($F = 6.76$; d.f. = 1, 14; $p < 0.05$), but not to the other subdimensions (anticipatory worry and pessimism: $F = 1.15$; d.f. = 1, 14; p = n.s.), fear of uncertainty ($F = 1.15$; d.f. = 1, 14; p = n.s.) and shyness with strangers ($F = 0.119$; d.f. = 1, 14; p = n.s.). Moreover, subjects with blunted CORT responses after IPS did not differ from nonblunted responders in any of the subdimensions (statistics not shown). Means and standard errors of personality dimensions according to each challenge study and response classification are given in figure 4.

Finally, the last question addressed was to compare subjects with blunted responses to both drugs with all the other participants of both studies. This classification yielded 6 subjects (blunted PRL responses after D-FEN and blunted CORT responses after IPS) against 10 subjects (blunted in one of the two or high responses in both studies). With respect to the subdimensions of HA it can clearly be seen in figure 5 that, given the adjusted level of significance (0.05/4 = 0.0125), subjects with blunted responses after both challenges reveal higher levels in fatigability and asthenia than all the other groups. This differ-

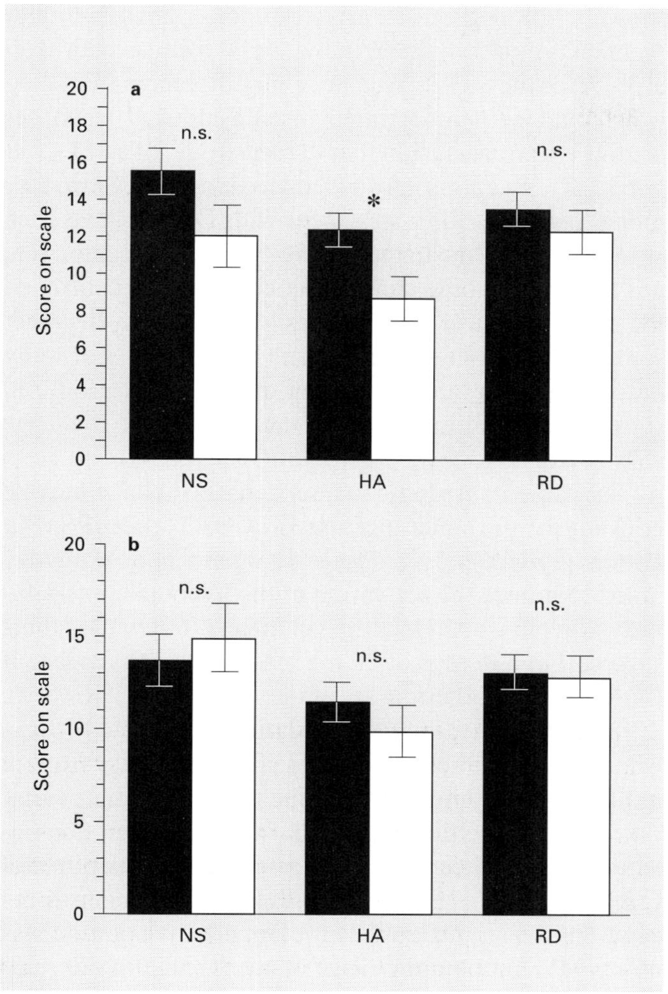

3

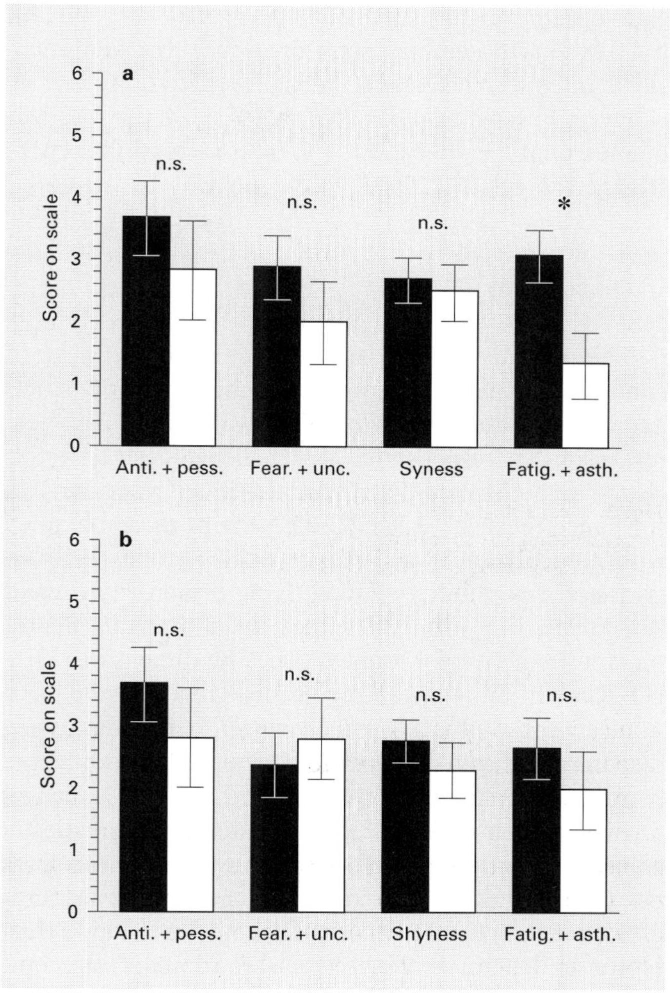

4

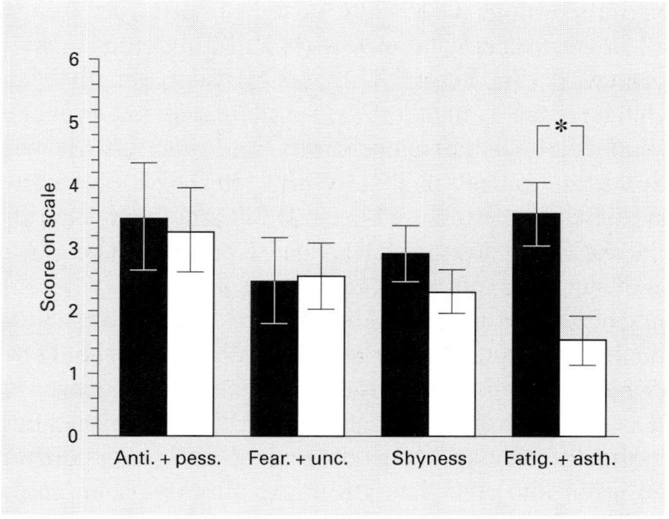

5

Fig. 3. Means ± SEM in the three major personality dimensions proposed by Cloninger according to the response classification for the D-FEN (**a**) and IPS (**b**) study (for statistics see text). ■ = Blunted; □ = increased. $^*p < 0.05$.

Fig. 4. Means ± SEM in subdimensions of HA according to the response classifications for the D-FEN (**a**) and IPS (**b**) study (for statistics see text). ■ = Blunted; □ = increased. $^*p < 0.05$.

Fig. 5. Means ± SEM in subdimensions of HA according to the response classification for the D-FEN and IPS study combined (for statistics see text). ■ = Blunted after both challenges (n = 6); □ = all others (n = 10). $^*p < 0.008$.

ence became highly significant ($F = 9.47$; d.f. = 1, 14; $p < 0.008$), while comparisons for all the other subdimensions failed to reach statistical significance (anticipatory worry and pessimism: $F = 0.03$; d.f. = 1, 14, p = n.s.; fear of uncertainty: $F = 0.01$; d.f. = 1, 14, p = n.s.; shyness with strangers: $F = 1.15$; d.f. = 1, 14, p = n.s.).

Discussion

The present studies were conducted to investigate if combined challenge paradigms may be superior to single approaches when relating personality dimensions to neurotransmitter responsivity by challenge tests. Results clearly demonstrated that a combination of responses to a substance releasing 5-HT (D-FEN) with those obtained with a highly specific 5-HT_{1a} partial agonist (IPS) increases the possibility of identifying personality dimensions related to hormonal indicators of a certain neurotransmitter activity. Moreover, specific dimensions of 5-HT-related traits (fatigability and asthenia) may be identified by the approach used. However, before discussing this aspect, a few remarks should be made concerning the two studies separately.

PRL responses to D-FEN were low but statistically highly significant (main effect not shown). The reason for lower responses may be seen in the unusually low dosage of 15 mg which was chosen to avoid unspecific stress responses due to side effects which are known for the commoner dosage of 30 mg (D-FEN) or 60 mg (*d-l*-fenfluramine) after which up to 90% of the subjects complained about headache, lightheadedness and difficulties in concentration [59]. Since PRL secretion has frequently been characterized as highly stress sensitive (e.g. [60–62]) one should carefully distinguish 5-HT- and/or stress (discomfort)-related effects on PRL. With 15 mg D-FEN, very few side effects were reported in our study. Another reason for the use of low doses of substances in personality research is the fact that individual differences in responsivity cannot be related to personality if all of the subjects show maximal responses. This possible ceiling effect should be avoided as well. However, others did not find changes in hormone concentrations in healthy subjects even after treatment with the 30 mg dose [63]. Several factors should be taken into consideration to explain these differences across studies which look quite similar in their design. On the one hand, characteristics of the subjects may be relevant. As has been described very recently, subjects practicing regular exercise differ in endocrine responses from their controls [64]. While CORT and PRL responses were shown to be reduced in athletes upon a challenge with meta-chlorophenylpiperazine, a 5-HT agonist with high affinity for the 5-HT_{2c} receptors, no differences from controls could be demonstrated for IPS-induced responses leading to the conclusion that the sensitivity of 5-HT_{2c} but not 5-HT_{1a} receptors may be reduced by sports. Since hormonal responses after treatment with D-FEN have been suggested to be mediated by the 5-$HT_{2a/2c}$ receptor [65, 66] the amount of exercise practice should be controlled for this challenge paradigm as well. Moreover, other sources of variance may also result in differences of study outcomes. For example, time of day [67] or season [68] show differential influence on the outcome of challenge with D-FEN.

The same nonspecific factors described above may be relevant for the small increases in CORT after IPS. But also in another study, a dosage between 5 and 30 mg/day failed to induce the activation of the hypothalamus-pituitary-adrenal axis in healthy volunteers [69] while others suggest that a dosage of 20 mg may be a useful dosage if CORT and hypothermia are of interest [69, 70]. However, in the cited study, the drug was administered at 10 a.m., whereas our regimen started at 3 p.m. which may explain a different outcome, possibly due to the circadian variation of CORT. Other factors like age have been demonstrated to influence the size of temperature reduction and CORT increase [71]. With increasing age, responses became smaller in males while for females the opposite was observed. However, the range of age is small in our sample, but interestingly, subjects with blunted responses tended to be older than high responders (28.17 ± 4.71 vs. 25.00 ± 2.98; $p = 0.12$).

The number of studies relating challenge studies to personality factors is limited. However, as described in the introduction, some studies follow the idea of a possibility to extrapolate from psychopathology to a nonclinical dimension of disease-related personality traits. For example, Cleare and Bond [46] demonstrated that in healthy volunteers, only males high on aggressiveness as measured by the Buss-Durkee Hostility Inventory showed blunted CORT responses after 30 mg D-FEN, while PRL responses were not differently affected in males and females. The relationship between D-FEN responses and aggression/impulsivity has been reported by several authors. Moreover, blunted PRL responses after D-FEN were associated with a relatively high morbid risk of impulsive personality disorder traits in the first-degree relatives of patients with a diagnosis of a personality disorder [72]. Since the validity of questionnaire data may be lower than behavioral measurements of personality dimensions, it is remarkable that blunted PRL responses after D-FEN are associated with both sources of personality assessment [73]. Additionally, comparable approaches to the D-FEN challenge test by e.g. meta-chlorophenylpiperazine revealed similar correlations with personality dimensions [74].

However, blunted PRL responses have been demonstrated for subjects scoring high on depression scales as well. As indicated by Gerra et al. [75], sons of mothers with major depressive episodes yielded blunted CORT and PRL responses to D-FEN. Depressed patients with high lethality suicide attempts have been demonstrated to exhibit lower PRL responses after D-FEN than subjects with low lethality suicide attempts [76]. Moreover, depressed younger inpatients (irrespectively of suicide attempts) exhibited blunted PRL changes whereas older ($\geq$30 years) did not [77]. However, data on healthy subjects high on depressiveness (i.e. low satisfaction with life) are not available up to now. The same is true for studies using IPS.

Therefore, it seemed justified to turn to the depressive anxious cluster of personality traits as characterized by the Cloninger scale of HA.

The data of the present study reveals that HA obviously relates to the serotonin system and therefore confirms that part of the model of Cloninger. However, the combination of releasing/reuptake-inhibiting probes with those acting on specific receptors like IPS may be helpful to identify specific aspects of HA. Interestingly, the fact that subjects blunted in both responses were characterized by high levels of fatigability and asthenia (which can be seen as one of the major components of neuroticism) means that subjects with blunted responses after D-FEN cannot be assumed to exhibit high levels of 5-HT-related personality traits if they show high responses after a challenge with IPS. The same conclusion must be drawn for IPS, leading to the overall assumption that postsynaptic 5-$HT_{2a/2c}$ and 5-HT_{1a} receptor sensitivities may be down-regulated in healthy subjects high on fatigability and asthenia.

Taken together, neurotransmitter challenge tests seem to be a useful tool to discover the biological basis of personality, and there is some evidence that they may be more valid than a direct assessment of possible indicators like CSF 5-HIAA [78]. However, the selection of useful substances is one of the most crucial points in challenge studies [79]. For example, *d-l*-fenfluramine (more than D-FEN) was shown to affect catecholamines as indicated by changes in dopaminergic and noradrenergic metabolite concentrations [80]. Therefore, studies using substances with high specificity for one of the two 5-HT_2 receptor subtypes administered as isolated tests or in combination with highly specific 5-HT_{1a} partial agonists, like IPS or flesinoxan, are needed to identify the relations between 5-HT and personality in more detail.

References

1 Anderson GM, Mefford IN, Tolliver TJ, Riddle MA, Ocame DM, Leckman JF, Cohen DJ: Serotonin in human lumbar cerebrospinal fluid: A reassessment. Life Sci 1990;46:247–255.

2 Trulson ME: Dietary tryptophan does not alter the function of brain serotonin neurons. Life Sci 1985;37:1067–1072.

3 Stahl SM: Platelets as pharmacological models for the receptors and biochemistry for monoaminergic neurons; in Longenecker GL (ed): The Platelets: Physiology and Pharmacology. New York, Academic Press, 1985, pp 307–340.

4 De Clerck F, Xhonneux B, Leysen J, Janssen PAJ: Evidence for functional 5-HT2 receptor sites on human blood platelets. Biochem Pharmacol 1984;33:2807–2811.

5 Flament MF, Rapoport JL, Murphy DL, Berg CJ, Lake CR: Biochemical changes during clomipramine treatment of childhood obsessive-compulsive disorder. Arch Gen Psychiatry 1987;44:219–255.

6 Power AC, Cowen PJ: Neuroendocrine challenge tests: Assessment of 5-HT function in anxiety and depression. Mol Aspects Med 1992;13:205–220.

7 Coccaro EF, Kavoussi RJ: Neuropsychopharmacologic challenge in biological psychiatry. Clin Chem 1994;40:319–327.

8 Meltzer HY: Role of the serotonergic system in pituitary hormone secretion: The pharmacologic challenge paradigm in man; in Vanhoutte PM, Saxena PR, Paoletti R, Brunello N, Jackson AS (eds): Serotonin. From Cell Biology to Pharmacology and Therapeutics. Milano, Kluver Academic Publishers, 1990, pp 239–247.

9 Ryan ND, Birmaher B, Perel JM, Dahl RE, Meyer V, al Shabbout M, Iyengar S, Puig Antich J: Neuroendocrine response to *L*-5-hydroxytryptophan challenge in prepubertal major depression. Depressed vs normal children. Arch Gen Psychiatry 1992;49:843–851.

10 Meltzer HY, Wiita B, Tricou BJ, Simonovic M, Fang V, Manov G: Effect of serotonin precursors and serotonin agonists on plasma hormone levels. Adv Biochem Psychopharmacol 1982; 34:117-139.

11 Pitchot W, Ansseau M, Gonzalez Moreno A, Lembreghts M, Hansenne M, Wauthy J, Reel C, Jammaer R, Papart P, Sulon J, Legros JJ: The flesinoxan 5-HT1A receptor challenge in major depression and suicidal behavior. Pharmacopsychiatry 1995;28:91–92.

12 Lopez Ibor JJ Jr, Saiz Ruiz J, Iglesias LM: The fenfluramine challenge test in the affective spectrum: A possible marker of endogeneity and severity. Pharmacopsychiatry 1988;21:9–14.

13 Cowen PJ: Serotonin receptor subtypes in depression: Evidence from studies in neuroendocrine regulation. Clin Neuropharmacol 1993; 16(suppl 3):S6–S18.

14 Stahl SM: Neuroendocrine markers of serotonin responsivity in depression. Prog Neuropsychopharmacol Biol Psychiatry 1992;16:655–659.
15 Rubin RT, Poland RE, Lesser IM, Martin DJ: Neuroendocrine aspects of primary endogenous depression. V. Serum prolactin measures in patients and matched control subjects. Biol Psychiatry 1989;25:4–21.
16 Van de Kar LD: Neuroendocrine aspects of the serotonergic hypothesis of depression. Neurosci Biobehav Rev 1989;13:237–246.
17 Cowen PJ, Charig EM: Neuroendocrine responses to intravenous tryptophan in major depression. Arch Gen Psychiatry 1987;44:958–966.
18 Atkinson JH Jr, Kremer EF, Risch SC, Dana R, Janowsky DS: Neuroendocrine responses in psychiatric and pain patients with major depression. Biol Psychiatry 1986;21:612–620.
19 Van Praag HM: Neuroendocrine disorders in depressions and their significance for the monoamine hypothesis of depression. Acta Psychiatr Scand 1978;57:389–404.
20 Deakin JF, Pennell I, Upadhyaya AJ, Lofthouse R: A neuroendocrine study of 5HT function in depression: Evidence for biological mechanisms of endogenous and psychosocial causation. Psychopharmacology (Berl) 1990; 101:85–92.
21 Coccaro EF: Central serotonin and impulsive aggression. Br J Psychiatry Suppl 1989;52–62.
22 Coccaro EF: Impulsive aggression and central serotonergic system function in humans: An example of a dimensional brain-behavior relationship. Int Clin Psychopharmacol 1992;7:3–12.
23 Stein DJ, Towey J, Hollander E: The neuropsychiatry of impulsive aggression; in Hollander E, Stein DJ (eds): Impulsivity and Aggression. Chichester, Wiley, 1995, pp 91–105.
24 Fineberg NA, Cowen PJ, Kirk JW, Montgomery SA: Neuroendocrine responses to intravenous *L*-tryptophan in obsessive compulsive disorder. J Affective Disord 1994;32:97–104.
25 Goodman WK, McDougle CJ, Price LH, Barr LC, Hills OF, Caplik JF, Charney DS, Heninger GR: *m*-Chlorophenylpiperazine in patients with obsessive-compulsive disorder: Absence of symptom exacerbation. Biol Psychiatry 1995;38:138–149.
26 af Klinteberg B, Schalling D, Edman G, Oreland L, Asberg M: Personality correlates of platelet monoamine oxidase (MAO) activity in female and male subjects. Neuropsychobiology 1987;18:89-96.
27 Schalling D, Edman G, Asberg M, Oreland L: Platelet MAO activity associated with impulsivity and aggressivity. Person Individ Diff 1988;9:597–605.
28 Coursey RD, Buchsbaum MS, Murphy DL: Psychological characteristics of subjects identified by platelet MAO activity and evoked potentials as biologically at risk for psychopathology. J Abnorm Psychol 1980;89:151–164.
29 Faustman WO, King RJ, Faull KF, Moses JA Jr, Benson KL, Zarcone VP, Csernansky JG: MMPI measures of impulsivity and depression correlate with CSF 5-HIAA and HVA in depression but not schizophrenia. J Affective Disord 1991;22:235–239.
30 Linnoila VM, Virkkunen M: Aggression, suicidality, and serotonin. J Clin Psychiatry 1992; 53(suppl):46–51.
31 Fishbein DH, Lozovsky D, Jaffe JH: Impulsivity, aggression, and neuroendocrine responses to serotonergic stimulation in substance abusers. Biol Psychiatry 1989;25:1049–1066.
32 Thakore JH, O'Keane V, Dinan TG: d-Fenfluramine-induced prolactin responses in mania: Evidence for serotonergic subsensitivity. Am J Psychiatry 1996;153:1460–1463.
33 Yatham LN: Prolactin and cortisol responses to fenfluramine challenge in mania. Biol Psychiatry 1996;39:285–288.
34 Cleare AJ, Murray RM, O'Keane V: Reduced prolactin and cortisol responses to *d*-fenfluramine in depressed compared to healthy matched control subjects. Neuropsychopharmacology 1996;14:349–354.
35 Maes M, D'Hondt P, Suy E, Minner B, Vandervorst C, Raus J: HPA-axis hormones and prolactin responses to dextro-fenfluramine in depressed patients and healthy controls. Prog Neuropsychopharmacol Biol Psychiatry 1991; 15:781–790.
36 O'Keane V, Dinan TG: Prolactin and cortisol responses to *d*-fenfluramine in major depression: Evidence for diminished responsivity of central serotonergic function. Am J Psychiatry 1991;148:1009–1015.
37 Newman ME, Shapria B, Lerer B: Evaluation of central serotonergic function in affective and related disorder by the fenfluramine challenge test: A critical review. Int J Neuropharmacol 1998;1:49–69.
38 Pitchot W, Ansseau M, Gonzalez Moreno A, Lembreghts M, Hansenne M, Wauthy J, Reel C, Jammaer R, Papart P, Sulon J, et al : The flesinoxan 5-HT1A receptor challenge in major depression and suicidal behavior. Pharmacopsychiatry 1995;28(suppl 2):91–92.
39 Meltzer HY, Maes M: Effects of buspirone on plasma prolactin and cortisol levels in major depressed and normal subjects. Biol Psychiatry 1994;35:316–323.
40 Cowen PJ, Anderson IM, Grahame Smith DG: Neuroendocrine effects of azapirones. J Clin Psychopharmacol 1990;10:21S–25S.
41 Meltzer HY, Maes M: Effects of ipsapirone on plasma cortisol and body temperature in major depression. Biol Psychiatry 1995;38:450–457.
42 Lesch KP, Mayer S, Disselkamp Tietze J, Hoh A, Wiesmann M, Osterheider M, Schulte HM: 5-HT1A receptor responsivity in unipolar depression. Evaluation of ipsapirone-induced ACTH and cortisol secretion in patients and controls. Biol Psychiatry 1990;28:620–628.
43 Shiah IS, Yatham LN, Lam RW, Tam EM, Zis AP: Cortisol, hypothermic, and behavioral responses to ipsapirone in patients with bipolar depression and normal controls. Neuropsychobiology 1998;38:6–12.
44 Lesch KP, Hoh A, Disselkamp Tietze J, Wiesmann M, Osterheider M, Schulte HM:5-Hydroxytryptamine1A receptor responsivity in obsessive-compulsive disorder. Comparison of patients and controls. Arch Gen Psychiatry 1991;48:540–547.
45 Coccaro EF, Kavoussi RJ, Hauger RL: Physiological responses to *d*-fenfluramine and ipsapirone challenge correlate with indices of aggression in males with personality disorder. Int Clin Psychopharmacol 1995;10:177–179.
46 Cleare AJ, Bond AJ: Does central serotonergic function correlate inversely with aggression? A study using *D*-fenfluramine in healthy subjects. Psychiatry Res 1997;69:89–95.
47 Netter P, Hennig J, Roed IS: Serotonin and dopamine as mediators of sensation seeking behavior. Neuropsychobiology 1996;34:155–165.
48 Netter P, Hennig J, Rohrmann S, Wyhlidal K, Hain-Herrmann M: Modification of experimentally induced aggression by temperament dimensions. Person Individ Diff 1998;25:873–887.
49 Cloninger CR: A unified biosocial theory of personality and its role in the development of anxiety states: A reply to commentaries. Psychiatr Dev 1988;2:83–120.
50 Nelson EC, Cloninger CR, Przybeck TR, Csernansky JG: Platelet serotonergic markers and Tridimensional Personality Questionnaire measures in a clinical sample. Biol Psychiatry 1996;40:271–278.
51 Pfohl B, Black D, Noyes R Jr, Kelley M, Blum N: A test of the tridimensional personality theory: Association with diagnosis and platelet imipramine binding in obsessive-compulsive disorder. Biol Psychiatry 1990;28:41–46.
52 Davies D, Dunlop SR, Shea P, Brittain H, Hendrie HC: Biological stress responses in high and low trait anxious students. Biol Psychiatry 1985;20:843–851.
53 Netter P: Serotonin reuptake inhibitors in healthy human subjects. Adv Biol Psychiatry 1988;17:31–46.
54 McTravish D, Heel RC: Dexfenfluramine. A review of its pharmacological properties and therapeutic potential in obesity. Arch Gen Psychiatry 1992;44:573–588.
55 Hennig J, Becker H, Netter P: 5-HT agonist-induced changes in peripheral immune cells in healthy volunteers: The impact of personality. Behav Brain Res 1996;73:359–363.
56 Lesch KP, Rupprecht R, Poten B, Muller U, Sohnle K, Fritze J, Schulte HM: Endocrine responses to 5-hydroxytryptamine-1A receptor activation by ipsapirone in humans. Biol Psychiatry 1989;26:203–205.
57 Cloninger CR: A systematic method for clinical description and classification of personality variants. A proposal. Arch Gen Psychol 1987; 44:573–588.

58 Weyers P, Krebs H, Janke W: Reliability and construct validity of the German version of Cloninger's tridimensional personality questionnaire. Person Individ Diff 1995;19:853–861.
59 Muldoon MF, Manuck SB, Jansma CL, Moore AL, Perel J, Mann JJ: *D,L*-fenfluramine challenge test: Experience in nonpatient sample. Biol Psychiatry 1996;39:761–768.
60 Armario A, Marti O, Molina T, de Pablo J, Valdes M: Acute stress markers in humans: Response of plasma glucose, cortisol and prolactin to two examinations differing in the anxiety they provoke. Psychoneuroendocrinology 1996;21:17–24.
61 Brooks JE, Herbert M, Walder CP, Selby C, Jeffcoate WJ: Prolactin and stress: Some endocrine correlates of pre-operative anxiety. Clin Endocrinol (Oxf) 1986;24:653–656.
62 Meyerhoff JL, Oleshansky MA, Mougey EH: Psychologic stress increases plasma levels of prolactin, cortisol, and POMC-derived peptides in man. Psychosom Med 1988;50:295–303.
63 Goodwin GM, Murray CL, Bancroft J: Oral *D*-fenfluramine and neuroendocrine challenge: problems with the 30 mg dose in men. J Affective Disord 1994;30:117–122.
64 Brooks A, Meyer T, George G, Hillmer-Vogel U, Meyer D, Bandelow B, Hajak G, Bartmann U, Gleiter CH, Ruether E: Decreased neuroendocrine responses to meta-chlorphenylpiperazine (mCPP) but normal responses to ipsapirone in marathon runners. Neuropsychopharmacology 1999;20:150–161.
65 Goodall EM, Cowen PJ, Franklin M, Silverstone T: Ritanserin attenuates anorectic, endocrine and thermic responses to *d*-fenfluramine in human volunteers. Psychopharmacology 1993;112:461–466.
66 Coccaro EF, Kavoussi RJ, Oakes M, Cooper TB, Hauger R: 5-HT 2a/2c receptor blockade by amesergide fully attenuates prolactin response to *d*-fenfluramine challenge in physically healthy human subjects. Psychopharmacology 1996;126:24–30.
67 Monteleone P, Bortolotti F, Orazzo C, Serino I, Maj M: Differences between morning and afternoon hormonal responses to *D*-fenfluramine in healthy humans. Psychoneuroendocrinology 1997;22:79–87.
68 Monteleone P, La Rocca A, Fuschino A, Bortolotti F, Maj M: Seasonal variation in plasma prolactin response to *d*-fenfluramine in healthy subjects. Psychoneuroendocrinology 1999;24:201–208.
69 Beneke M, Wingender W, Horstmann R, Konrad Dalhoff I, Weber H, Kuhlmann J, Schmidt BH: Neuroendocrine effects of ipsapirone on the hypothalamic-pituitary adrenal axis: CRF, ACTH and cortisol in healthy volunteers. Eur J Clin Pharmacol 1992;42:163–169.
70 Kahn RS, Trestman R, Lawlor BA, Gabriel S, Davidson M, Siever L: Effects of ipsapirone in healthy subjects: A dose-response study. Psychopharmacology (Berl) 1994;114:155–160.
71 Gelfin Y, Lerer B, Lesch KP, Gorfine M, Allolio B: Complex effects of age and gender on hypothermic, adrenocorticotrophic hormone and cortisol responses to ipsapirone challenge in normal subjects. Psychopharmacology (Berl) 1995;120:356–364.
72 Coccaro EF, Silverman JM, Klar HM, Horvath TB, Siever LJ: Familial correlates of reduced central serotonergic system function in patients with personality disorders. Arch Gen Psychiatry 1994;51:318–324.
73 Coccaro EF, Berman ME, Kavoussi RJ, Hauger RL: Relationship of prolactin response to *d*-fenfluramine to behavioral and questionnaire assessments of aggression in personality-disordered men (see comments). Biol Psychiatry 1996;40:157–164.
74 Coccaro EF, Kavoussi RJ, Trestman RL, Gabriel SM, Cooper TB, Siever LJ: Serotonin function in human subjects: Intercorrelations among central 5-HT indices and aggressiveness. Psychiatry Res 1997;73:1–14.
75 Gerra G, Caccavari R, Zaimovic A, Palladino M, Chittolini B, Giucastro G, Maestri D, Monica C, Fertonani Affini G, Delsignore R, Brambilla F: Serotonergic function in mothers of opioid addicts: Correlation with comorbid depression. Acta Psychiatr Scand 1997;96:36–42.
76 Malone KM, Corbitt EM, Li S, Mann JJ: Prolactin response to fenfluramine and suicide attempt lethality in major depression. Br J Psychiatry 1996;168:324–329.
77 Mann JJ, McBride PA, Malone KM, DeMeo M, Keilp J: Blunted serotonergic responsivity in depressed inpatients. Neuropsychopharmacology 1995;13:53–64.
78 Coccaro EF, Kavoussi RJ, Cooper TB, Hauger RL: Central serotonin activity and aggression: Inverse relationship with prolactin response to *d*-fenfluramine, but not CSF 5-HIAA concentration, in human subjects. Am J Psychiatry 1997;154:1430–1435.
79 Yatham LN, Steiner M: Neuroendocrine probes of serotonergic function: A critical review. Life Sci 1993;53:447–463.
80 Mitchell PB, Smythe GA: Endocrine and amine responses to *D,L*-fenfluramine in normal subjects. Psychiatry Res 1991;39:141–153.

Neuropsychobiology

Neuropsychobiology 2000;41:48–53

An Interaction between the Catechol O-Methyltransferase and Serotonin Transporter Promoter Region Polymorphisms Contributes to Tridimensional Personality Questionnaire Persistence Scores in Normal Subjects

Jonathan Benjamin[a] Yamima Osher[a] Pesach Lichtenberg[b] Rachel Bachner-Melman[b] Inga Gritsenko[b] Moshe Kotler[c] Robert H. Belmaker[c] Vadim Valsky[b] Michael Drendel[b] Richard P. Ebstein[b]

[a]Faculty of Health Sciences, Ben Gurion University of the Negev, Beersheva, [b]Research Laboratory, S. Herzog Memorial Hospital Israel, Jerusalem, and [c]Beersheva Mental Health Center, Faculty of Health Sciences, Ben-Gurion University of the Negev, Beersheva, Israel

Key Words

Tridimensional Personality Questionnaire · Persistence · Catechol O-methyltransferase · Serotonin transporter promoter region · Polymorphism · Personality · Genes

Abstract

Persistence (RD2) is a subscale of the reward dependence trait, one of the three major personality factors assessed by the Tridimensional Personality Questionnaire (TPQ). Subjects with high RD2 scores are characterized as industrious, hard-working, ambitious, perfectionistic. TPQ scores were examined in 577 normal subjects inventoried for two common genetic polymorphisms, the catechol O-methyltransferase (COMT) valine to methionine (val to met) amino acid substitution that determines high and low enzyme activity, and the serotonin transporter promoter region 44 bp deletion (5-HTTLPR) linked in some studies to harm avoidance or neuroticism. When TPQ RD2 scores are grouped by COMT and 5-HTTLPR polymorphisms and analyzed by two-way ANOVA, significant main effects for COMT ($F = 2.98$, $p = 0.05$) and 5-HTTLPR ($F = 4.27$, $p = 0.04$) and a significant interaction COMT × 5-HTTLPR ($F = 6.18$, $p = 0.002$) are observed. In the presence of COMT homozygosity (val/val or met/met genotypes), the presence of the short 5-HTTLPR allele raises RD2 scores. The effect of these two polymorphisms on RD2 was also examined using a within-families design. Siblings in our data set who shared identical genotypes had significantly correlated RD2 scores (intraclass coefficient = 0.34, $F = 2.03$, $p = 0.002$, $n = 67$), whereas sibs with dissimilar genotypes in at least one polymorphism showed no significant correlation for RD2 scores (intraclass coefficient = 0.105, $F = 1.23$, $p = 0.16$, $n = 92$).

Introduction

The Tridimensional Personality Questionnaire (TPQ) is a 100-question self-report instrument that originally discriminated between three major personality traits [1]. High scorers on novelty seeking (NS) can be characterized as exploratory, curious, impulsive, extravagant; on harm avoidance (HA) as worrying and pessimistic, fearful, shy, fatigable; on reward dependence (RD) as sentimental, dedicated, dependent. More recently, persistence (RD2, a

KARGER

Fax + 41 61 306 12 34
E-Mail karger@karger.ch
www.karger.com

0302–282X/00/0411–0048$17.50/0

Accessible online at:
www.karger.com/journals/nps

Prof. Richard P. Ebstein
Research Laboratory, S. Herzog Memorial Hospital
PO Box 35300
Jerusalem 91351 (Israel)
Tel. +972 2 5316853, Fax +972 2 5316853, E-Mail ebstein@netmedia.net.il

subscale of RD) was suggested as a separate trait, and such individuals are defined as industrious, hard-working, ambitious, perfectionistic. Twin studies [2, 3] demonstrate a significant heritable component to personality factors measured by various questionnaires, but only recently have specific genes been associated with such traits [4, 5].

Catechol O-methyltransferase (COMT) along with monoamine oxidase is one of the two enzymes that account for the first steps in the elimination of catecholamines [6]. The physiological substrates of COMT include dopamine, norepinephrine and adrenaline, but in contrast to monoamine oxidase, serotonin is not a substrate for this enzyme [7]. A common COMT coding for a thermolabile low-activity enzyme has been recognized for two decades [8]. A single amino acid substitution (valine to methionine, val108/met) in exon IV accounts for differences in thermolability: val/val homozygotes display high, val/met intermediate and met/met 4–5 times lower COMT activity [9].

Several recent studies indicate a role of COMT in obsessive-compulsive disorder [10–13]. This enzyme has also been implicated in impulsive behavior in schizophrenic subjects [14–16], in children with attention deficit hyperactivity disorder [17] and in polysubstance abuse [18]. These studies suggested to us that COMT might contribute not only to abnormal behavior, but also to normal human personality traits. Heils et al. [19] and Lesch et al. [20] recently reported an association between anxiety-related traits such as NEO neuroticism and TPQ HA with a newly described functional polymorphism in the serotonin transporter transcriptional control region (5-HTTLPR). The short version of the promoter region contains a 44-bp deletion that results in reduced mRNA transcription and reduced levels of serotonin transporter. In the current study, we simultaneously examined both of these functional polymorphisms, COMT and 5-HTTLPR, for their association with TPQ personality scores, by two-way ANOVA.

Method

Subject Groups

There were 240 males and 337 females; average age was 27.9 (10.84 SD). Subjects were recruited from many sources (high schools, villages, kibbutz members, university students and staff) and paid for their participation in the study. No psychiatric screening was carried out, but the sib pairs were asked about a history of mental illness and substance abuse (data will be presented elsewhere). About 50% of the subjects were related sib pairs. The Ben-Gurion University Helsinki Human Subjects Committee approved the study.

Table 1. TPQ RD2 scores grouped by the COMT and 5-HTTLPR polymorphisms

5-HTTLPR	COMT	Mean	SD	n
l/l	val/val high activity	4.43	2.10	42
	val/met heterozygote	5.38	1.82	84
	met/met low activity	3.95	2.53	19
s/l and s/s	val/val high activity	5.40	2.21	129
	val/met	4.95	2.06	209
	met/met low activity	4.94	2.13	94

Total n = 577.

TPQ Persistence

In the current study, a Hebrew version of the TPQ was employed. In its initial version, the TPQ defined three major personality traits and included four subscales for each trait [1]. Cloninger subsequently defined subscale 2 (RD2) of the reward dependence dimension as persistence. In the current study, the original TPQ was employed and not the Temperament Character Index [21].

Genotyping

DNA was extracted and genotypes determined as previously described 5-HTTLPR [22] and COMT [23].

Statistical Analysis

All statistical analyses were carried out using SPSS for Windows. The effect of genotype on personality factors was examined by two-way ANOVA with sex as a covariate. Subsequent tests were also carried out using ANOVA with sex as a covariate. In the ANOVA analysis there were three levels for the COMT polymorphism: val/val, val/met and met/met. Principal analyses of the effect of the 5-HTTLPR polymorphism were performed after grouping the genotypes according to the short version (s/s and s/l) vs. the long version (l/l), i.e. assuming a dominant effect of the short allele validated by Lesch et al. [20] by in vitro experiments.

Results

When TPQ RD2 scores are grouped by COMT and 5-HTTLPR polymorphisms and analyzed by two-way ANOVA (RD2 is the dependent variable and COMT and 5-HTTLPR are the independent variables), significant main effects for COMT ($F = 2.98$, $p = 0.05$) and 5-HTTLPR ($F = 4.27$, $p = 0.04$) and a significant interaction COMT × 5-HTTLPR ($F = 6.18$, $p = 0.002$) are observed. Mean TPQ RD2 scores for the 577 subjects grouped by the two genotypes (5-HTTLPR and COMT) are summarized in table 1. In order to illustrate the interaction between these two polymorphisms, mean RD2 scores grouped by both polymorphisms are shown in figure 1. In

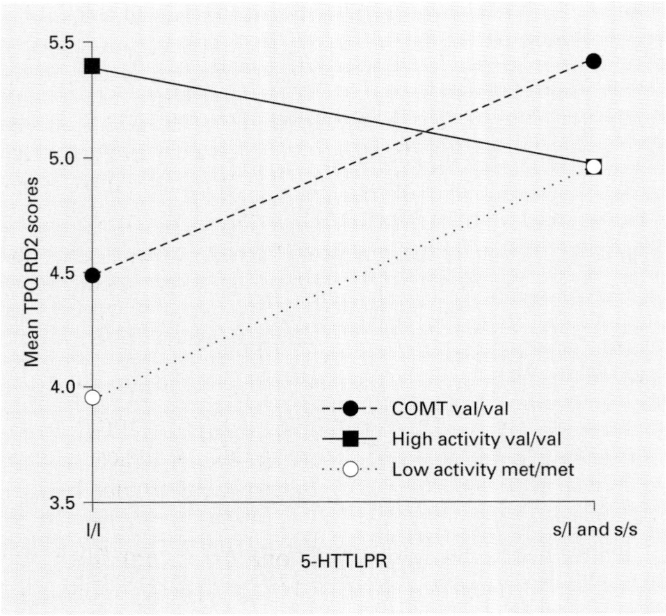

Fig. 1. TPQ RD2 scores grouped by the COMT and 5-HTTLPR polymorphisms. l/l = 5-HTTLPR long genotype; s/s and s/l = 5-HTTLPR short genotypes. The left y-axis groups subjects with the l/l 5-HTTLPR genotype and the right y-axis groups subjects with either the s/l or s/s 5-HTTLPR genotype. The three lines represent the three COMT genotypes and indicate how the two polymorphisms interact.

the presence of COMT homozygosity (val/val or met/met genotypes) the presence of the short 5-HTTLPR allele raises RD2 scores. No significant main effects or interactions were observed between the three major TPQ personality factors (NS, HA and RD total score) and COMT and 5-HTTLPR.

When subjects are selected for COMT val/val homozygosity, a significant ($F = 5.54$, $p = 0.02$) mean difference in RD2 scores is observed between subjects with the 5-HTTLPR s/s and s/l genotypes (RD2 mean score = 5.4, SD = 2.21, n = 129) and the l/l genotype (RD2 mean score = 4.43, SD = 2.1, n = 42). When subjects were selected for the COMT met/met genotype, a difference in RD2 scores is also observed between subjects with the 5-HTTLPR s/s and s/l genotypes (RD2 mean score = 4.94, SD = 2.13, n = 94) and the l/l genotype (RD2 mean score = 3.95, SD = 2.53, n = 19). However, this difference is only marginally significant ($F = 3.39$, $p = 0.07$).

The subjects we genotyped represent two independently recruited groups. We therefore examined the association between COMT and 5-HTTLPR in each of these sets. A significant interaction between COMT × 5-HTTLPR was observed both in the Beersheva set ($F = 2.83$, $p = 0.06$, $n = 209$) and in the Jerusalem set ($F = 3.71$, $p = 0.03$, $n = 368$).

Finally, we also examined the COMT × 5-HTTLPR interaction in a group of 159 siblings in our data set. In the 67 siblings with identical genotypes (COMT and 5-HTTLPR), a significant intraclass correlation for RD2 scores (coefficient = 0.34, $F = 2.03$, $p = 0.002$, $n = 67$) was observed. Conversely, in siblings with nonidentical genotypes for either the COMT or 5-HTTLPR genotypes, no significant intraclass correlation in RD2 scores (coefficient = 0.105, $F = 1.23$, $p = 0.16$, $n = 92$) was observed.

Discussion

The main finding of the present investigation is that an interaction between two functional polymorphisms, COMT and 5-HTTLPR, contributes to the determination of TPQ RD2 scores in a large group of 577 subjects. The short allele of the serotonin transporter raises RD2 scores in individuals homozygous for the COMT polymorphism. At the neurochemical level the present study suggests that homozygosity at COMT coupled with increased serotonin levels raises TPQ RD2 scores. From a psychological perspective, TPQ RD2 scores, including perfectionism and traits closely related to 'Type A' personality, are higher in the presence of a polymorphism (the 5-HTTLPR short allele) associated in some studies [20] with a personality factor characterized by high HA or neuroticism.

The COMT polymorphism examined in the current study, like many common variants of human genes, differs in allele frequency across ethnic and population groups [24, 25] Ethnic differences in allele frequency are a potential source of type I and type II errors in case-control association studies, and we therefore used the sib pairs in this data set to further examine the simultaneous effect of these three polymorphisms on RD2 scores. Sibs who shared identical genotypes for both polymorphisms showed a significant correlation in RD2 scores, whereas sibs having at least one dissimilar polymorphism showed no significant correlation in RD2 scores. These results suggest that ethnic stratification is not an explanation for the current findings.

Although it is seemingly counterintuitive that homozygosity for both met/met and val/val COMT genotypes interacts similarly with the 5-HTTLPR polymorphism to raise TPQ RD2 scores, this observation may be understandable in the light of other recent investigations showing a pleiotropic role of this gene on behavior [25, 26]. For example, both COMT val/val and met/met genotypes have been connected to disturbances in impulse control, as observed in attention deficit hyperactivity disorder (val/val genotype) [23], polysubstance abuse (val/val) [18] and violence (met/met) [14–16]. Thus, a phenotype shared across clinical nosologies and characterized by a similar impairment in executive control is associated with both COMT homozygous genotypes. A second example demonstrating that homozygosity for either genotype in a biallelic polymorphism may partially determine the same phenotype is provided by two recent meta-analyses that examined the role of the dopamine D3 receptor (DRD3) polymorphism in schizophrenia [27, 28]. Williams et al. [28] performed a meta-analysis of over 30 case-control studies of the association between schizophrenia and the *Bal*I polymorphism in exon 1 of the DRD3 gene. They observed a significant excess of both forms of homozygosity in patients (p = 0.0009) in their very large combined sample of over 5,000 individuals. Regarding the DRD3, it is interesting that an association has also recently been observed between homozygosity at both alleles and opiate dependence [29].

We cannot attribute the effects of the COMT polymorphism to a particular catecholaminergic neurotransmitter nor to a particular anatomical region. Noradrenaline, dopamine and adrenaline are all substrates for COMT, and each of these three catecholamines has important roles in mediating behavior in man. The broad substrate specificity of COMT and its distribution in both neuronal and nonneuronal cells [30] in various brain areas [31–34] confounds our attempts at the present time to determine more exactly the particular neurochemical and neuroanatomical pathways involved in the contribution of this enzyme to enhancing complex behavioral phenotypes such as observed in the current study.

The current results are also relevant to a recent report associating the low enzyme activity COMT met/met genotype with obsessive-compulsive disorder, especially in male subjects [11, 13]. Obsessive-compulsive disorder might be considered an extreme outcome of the normal RD2 personality trait (= industrious, hard-working, ambitious, perfectionist). Moreover, some unpublished observations suggest that obsessive-compulsive disorder patients and their unaffected relatives score high on TPQ RD2 [Ada Zohar, pers. commun.].

In the current investigation, we fail to replicate the original observation of Lesch et al. [20] regarding the association between anxiety or HA and the 5-HTTLPR short allele. Indeed, several previous reports [35–38], including one from our own group [22], have not observed this relationship. Nevertheless, as we discussed extensively in a recent publication [39], and based on two previous studies from our group [40, 41], we observed an indirect effect of the serotonin transporter and HA apparently mediated by an interaction between the 5-HTTLPR and the dopamine D4 receptor (DRD4) exon III repeat polymorphisms. This interaction has been observed in 2-week-old neonates [41], in the same children assessed again at 2 months of age [40] and in adults. In both infants and adults, short alleles of 5-HTTLPR and long alleles of DRD4 opposed each other's effects; i.e. approach behaviors (orientation to environmental stimuli in infants and NS in adults) are promoted by long DRD4 alleles, whereas short alleles of 5-HTTLPR increase avoidance behaviors.

The current investigation is one of several from our own [39–42] and other centers [43–45] that demonstrate the importance of examining multiple interactions between common genetic polymorphisms in order to more completely understand the role of genes in contributing to personality factors. In the first genome-wide scan [46] to search for loci contributing to TPQ personality factors, significant linkage was detected between HA and a locus on chromosome 8p21–23 that explained 38% of the trait variance. There was significant evidence of epistasis between the locus on 8p and others on chromosomes 18p, 20p and 21q. These interactions between various chromosomal linkage sites accounted for most of the genetic variance contributing to HA. There was also suggestive evidence of epistasis in other personality traits. Similarly, we [42] and a group in Germany [45] have provisional evidence that RD behavior is partially determined by at least two polymorphisms: the 5-HT2c receptor and the DRD4 exon III repeat region. The effect of these polymorphisms on personality may be quite broad, since the DRD4 not only contributes to reward and NS [4, 5], but also to HA as suggested by data from our own group [39] and that of Strobel [pers. commun.]. These pleiotropic effects of common polymorphisms on complex behavioral traits are not surprising, since most components of neural transmission including elements like receptors, transporters and enzymes are widely distributed in the brain and mutually modulate each other's activities and functions.

Acknowledgments

This research was supported in part by a grant by The Israel Science Foundation founded by the Israel Academy of Sciences and Humanities (R.P.E.).

References

1 Cloninger CR: A systematic method for clinical description and classification of personality variants. A proposal. Arch Gen Psychiatry 1987;44:573–588.

2 Bergeman CS, Chipuer HM, Plomin R, Pedersen NL, McClearn GE, Nesselroade JR, Costa PT Jr, McCrae RR: Genetic and environmental effects on openness to experience, agreeableness, and conscientiousness: An adoption/twin study. J Pers 1993;61:159–179.

3 Heath AC, Cloninger CR, Martin NG: Testing a model for the genetic structure of personality: A comparison of the personality systems of Cloninger and Eysenck. J Pers Soc Psychol 1994;66:762–775.

4 Benjamin J, Li L, Patterson C, Greenberg BD, Murphy DL, Hamer DH: Population and familial association between the D4 dopamine receptor gene and measures of Novelty Seeking. Nat Genet 1996;12:81–84.

5 Ebstein RP, Novick O, Umansky R, Priel B, Osher Y, Blaine D, Bennett ER, Nemanov L, Katz M, Belmaker RH: Dopamine D4 receptor (D4DR) exon III polymorphism associated with the human personality trait of Novelty Seeking. Nat Genet 1996;12:78–80.

6 Boulton AA, Eisenhofer G: Catecholamine metabolism. From molecular understanding to clinical diagnosis and treatment. Overview. Adv Pharmacol 1998;42:273–292.

7 Mannisto PT: Catechol O-methyltransferase: Characterization of the protein, its gene, and the preclinical pharmacology of COMT inhibitors. Adv Pharmacol 1998;42:324–328.

8 Weinshilboum R, Dunnette J: Thermal stability and the biochemical genetics of erythrocyte catechol-O-methyl-transferase and plasma dopamine-beta-hydroxylase. Clin Genet 1981;19:426–437.

9 Lachman HM, Papolos DF, Saito T, Yu YM, Szumlanski CL, Weinshilboum RM: Human catechol-O-methyltransferase pharmacogenetics: Description of a functional polymorphism and its potential application to neuropsychiatric disorders. Pharmacogenetics 1996;6:243–250.

10 Gogos JA, Morgan M, Luine V, Santha M, Ogawa S, Pfaff D, Karayiorgou M: Catechol-O-methyltransferase-deficient mice exhibit sexually dimorphic changes in catecholamine levels and behavior. Proc Natl Acad Sci USA 1998;95:9991–9996.

11 Karayiorgou M, Altemus M, Galke BL, Goldman D, Murphy DL, Ott J, Gogos JA: Genotype determining low catechol-O-methyltransferase activity as a risk factor for obsessive-compulsive disorder. Proc Natl Acad Sci USA 1997;94:4572–4575.

12 Karayiorgou M, Gogos JA, Galke BL, Wolyniec PS, Nestadt G, Antonarakis SE, Kazazian HH, Housman DE, Pulver AE: Identification of sequence variants and analysis of the role of the catechol-O-methyl-transferase gene in schizophrenia susceptibility. Biol Psychiatry 1998;43:425–431.

13 Karayiorgou M, Sobin C, Blundell ML, Galke BL, Malinova L, Goldberg P, Ott J, Gogos JA: Family-based association studies support a sexually dimorphic effect of COMT and MAOA on genetic susceptibility to obsessive-compulsive disorder (in process citation). Biol Psychiatry 1999;45:1178–1189.

14 Kotler M, Peretz B, Cohen H, Averbuch AV, Grinshpoon A, Gritsenko I, Nemanov L, Ebstein RP: Homicidal behavior in schizophrenia associated with a genetic polymorphism determining low catechol O-methyltransferase (COMT) activity. Am J Med Genet (Neuropsychiatr Genet), in press.

15 Lachman HM, Nolan KA, Mohr P, Saito T, Volavka J: Association between catechol O-methyltransferase genotype and violence in schizophrenia and schizoaffective disorder. Am J Psychiatry 1998;155:835–837.

16 Strous RD, Bark N, Parsia SS, Volavka J, Lachman HM: Analysis of a functional catechol-O-methyltransferase gene polymorphism in schizophrenia: Evidence for association with aggressive and antisocial behavior. Psychiatry Res 1997;69:71–77.

17 Eisenberg J, Zohar A, Mei-Tal G, Steinberg A, Tartakovsky E, Gritsenko I, Nemanov L, Ebstein RP: A haplotype relative risk study of the dopamine D4 receptor (DRD4) exon III repeat polymorphism and attention deficit hyperactivity disorder (ADHD). Am J Med Gen (Neuropsychiatr Genet), in press.

18 Vandenbergh DJ, Rodriguez LA, Miller IT, Uhl GR, Lachman HM: High-activity catechol-O-methyltransferase allele is more prevalent in polysubstance abusers. Am J Med Genet 1997;74:439–442.

19 Heils A, Teufel A, Petri S, Stober G, Riederer P, Bengel D, Lesch KP: Allelic variation of human serotonin transporter gene expression. J Neurochem 1996;66:2621–2624.

20 Lesch KP, Bengel D, Heils A, Sabol SZ, Greenberg BD, Petri S, Benjamin J, Muller CR, Hamer DH, Murphy DL: Association of anxiety-related traits with a polymorphism in the serotonin transporter gene regulatory region (see comments). Science 1996;274:1527–1531.

21 Cloninger CR, Svrakic DM, Przybeck TR: A psychobiological model of temperament and character. Arch Gen Psychiatry 1993;50:975–990.

22 Ebstein RP, Gritsenko I, Nemanov L, Frisch A, Osher Y, Belmaker RH: No association between the serotonin transporter gene regulatory region polymorphism and the Tridimensional Personality Questionnaire (TPQ) temperament of harm avoidance. Mol Psychiatry 1997;2:224–226.

23 Eisenberg J, Mei-Tal G, Steinberg A, Tartakovsky A, Gritsenko I, Nemanov L, Ebstein RP: A haplotype relative risk study of catechol-O-methyltransferase (COMT) and attention deficit hyperactivity disorder (ADHD): Association of the high-enzyme activity val allele with ADHD impulsive-hyperactive phenotype. Am J Med Genet (Neuropsychiatr Genet), in press.

24 Gelernter J, Cubells JF, Kidd JR, Pakstis AJ, Kidd KK: Population studies of polymorphisms of the serotonin transporter protein gene. Am J Med Genet 1999;88:61–66.

25 Kidd KK, Morar B, Castiglione CM, Zhao H, Pakstis AJ, Speed WC, Bonne-Tamir B, Lu RB, Goldman D, Lee C, Nam YS, Grandy DK, Jenkins T, Kidd JR: A global survey of haplotype frequencies and linkage disequilibrium at the DRD2 locus. Hum Genet 1998;103:211–227.

26 Lachman HM, Morrow B, Shprintzen R, Veit S, Parsia SS, Faedda G, Goldberg R, Kucherlapati R, Papolos DF: Association of codon 108/158 catechol-O-methyltransferase gene polymorphism with the psychiatric manifestations of velo-cardio-facial syndrome. Am J Med Genet 1996;67:468–472.

27 Dubertret C, Gorwood P, Ades J, Feingold J, Schwartz JC, Sokoloff P: Meta-analysis of DRD3 gene and schizophrenia: Ethnic heterogeneity and significant association in Caucasians. Am J Med Genet 1998;81:318–322.

28 Williams J, McGuffin P, Nothen M, Owen MJ: Meta-analysis of association between the 5-HT2a receptor T102C polymorphism and schizophrenia. EMASS Collaborative Group. European Multicentre Association Study of Schizophrenia (letter). Lancet 1997;349:1221.

29 Duaux E, Gorwood P, Griffon N, Bourdel MC, Sautel F, Sokoloff P, Schwartz JC, Ades J, Loo H, Poirier MF: Homozygosity at the dopamine D3 receptor gene is associated with opiate dependence (in process citation). Mol Psychiatry 1998;3:333–336.

30 Reenila I, Tuomainen P, Soinila S, Mannisto PT: Increase of catechol-O-methyltransferase activity in rat brain microglia after intrastriatal infusion of fluorocitrate, a glial toxin. Neurosci Lett 1997;230:155–158.

31 Hong J, Shu-Leong H, Tao X, Lap-Ping Y: Distribution of catechol-O-methyltransferase expression in human central nervous system (in process citation). Neuroreport 1998;9:2861–2864.

32 Karhunen T, Tilgmann C, Ulmanen I, Panula P: Catechol-O-methyltransferase (COMT) in rat brain: Immunoelectron microscopic study with an antiserum against rat recombinant COMT protein. Neurosci Lett 1995;187:57–60.

33 Karhunen T, Tilgmann C, Ulmanen I, Panula P: Neuronal and non-neuronal catechol-O-methyltransferase in primary cultures of rat brain cells. Int J Dev Neurosci 1995;13:825–834.

34 Karhunen T, Ulmanen I, Panula P: Catechol-O-methyltransferase in rat sensory ganglia and spinal cord. Neuroscience 1996;73:267–276.

35 Flory JD, Manuck SB, Ferrell RE, Dent KM, Peters DG, Muldoon MF: Neuroticism is not associated with the serotonin promoter (5-HTTLPR) polymorphism. Mol Psychiatry 1999;4:93–96.

36 Gelernter J, Kranzler H, Coccaro EF, Siever LJ, New AS: Serotonin transporter protein gene polymorphism and personality measures in African American and European American subjects. Am J Psychiatry 1998;155:1332–1338.
37 Gustavsson JP, Nothen MM, Jonsson EG, Neidt H, Forslund K, Rylander G, Mattila-Evenden M, Sedvall GC, Propping P, Asberg M: No association between serotonin transporter gene polymorphisms and personality traits. Neuropsychiatr Genet, submitted.
38 Jorm AF, Henderson AS, Jacomb PA, Christensen H, Korten AE, Rodgers B, Tan X, Easteal S: An association study of a functional polymorphism of the serotonin transporter with personality and psychiatric symptoms. Mol Psychiatry 1998;3:449–451.
39 Benjamin JYO, Kotler M, Gritsenko I, Nemanov L, Belmaker RH, Ebstein RP: TPQ personality trait of novelty seeking associated with the dopamine receptor D4 exon III (DRD4), serotonin transporter promoter region (5-HTTLPR) and catechol O-methyltransferase (COMT val-met) polymorphisms. Mol Psychiatry, in press.
40 Auerbach J, Geller V, Letzer S, Shinwell R, Belmaker RH, Levine J, Ebstein RP: Dopamine D4 receptor (D4DR) and serotonin transporter promoter (5-HTTLPR) polymorphisms in the determination of temperament in two month old infants. Mol Psychiatry 1999;4:369–373.
41 Ebstein RP, Levine J, Geller V, Auerbach J, Gritsenko I, Belmaker RH: Dopamine D4 receptor and serotonin transporter promoter in the determination of neonatal temperament. Mol Psychiatry 1998;3:238–246.
42 Ebstein RP, Segman R, Benjamin J, Osher Y, Nemanov L, Belmaker RH: 5-HT2C (HTR2C) serotonin receptor gene polymorphism associated with the human personality trait of reward dependence: Interaction with dopamine D4 receptor (D4DR) and dopamine D3 receptor (D3DR) polymorphisms. Am J Med Genet 1997;74:65–72.
43 Comings DE, Wu S, Chiu C, Ring RH, Gade R, Ahn C, MacMurray JP, Dietz G, Muhleman D: Polygenic inheritance of Tourette syndrome, stuttering, attention deficit hyperactivity, conduct, and oppositional defiant disorder: The additive and subtractive effect of the three dopaminergic genes – DRD2, D beta H, and DAT1. Am J Med Genet 1996;67:264–288.
44 Noble EP, Ozkaragoz TZ, Ritchie TL, Zhang X, Belin TR, Sparkes RS: D2 and D4 dopamine receptor polymorphisms and personality. Am J Med Genet 1998;81:257–267.
45 Kuhn KU, Meyer K, Nothen MM, Gansicke M, Papassotiropoulos A, Maier W: Allelic variants of dopamine receptor D4 (DRD4) and serotonin receptor 5HT2c (HTR2c) and temperament factors: Replication tests. Am J Med Genet 1999;88:168–172.
46 Cloninger CR, Van Eerdewegh P, Goate A, Edenberg HJ, Blangero J, Hesselbrock V, Reich T, Nurnberger J Jr, Schuckit M, Porjesz B, Crowe R, Rice JP, Foroud T, Przybeck TR, Almasy L, Bucholz K, Wu W, Shears S, Carr K, Crose C, Willig C, Zhao J, Tischfield JA, Li TK, Conneally PM: Anxiety proneness linked to epistatic loci in genome scan of human personality traits. Am J Med Genet 1998;81:313–317.

Neuropsychobiology

Author Index Vol. 41, No. 1, 2000

Subject Index Vol. 41, No. 1, 2000

KARGER
Fax + 41 61 306 12 34
E-Mail karger@karger.ch
www.karger.com

Accessible online at:
www.karger.com/journals/nps

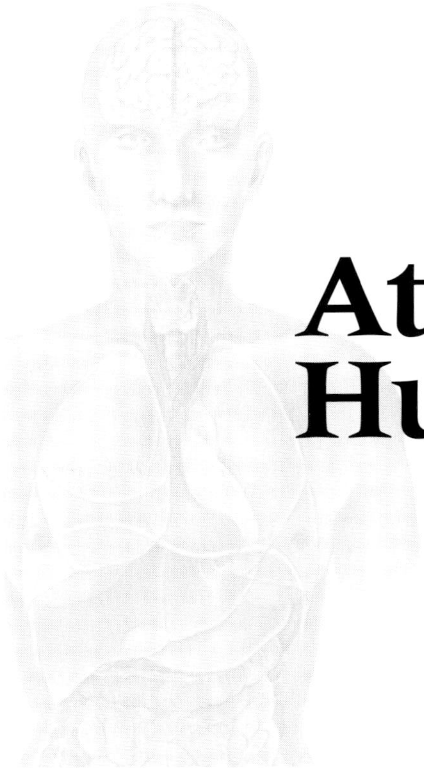